FAMILY TROUBLE

FAMILY TROUBLE

Middle-Class Parents, Children's Problems, and the Disruption of Everyday Life

ARA FRANCIS

RUTGERS UNIVERSITY PRESS
New Brunswick, New Jersey, and London

Library of Congress Cataloging-in-Publication Data

Francis, Ara.
Family trouble : middle-class parents, children's problems, and the disruption of
everyday life / Ara Francis.
pages cm
Includes bibliographical references and index.
ISBN 978-0-8135-7053-2 (hardcover : alk. paper)—ISBN 978-0-8135-7052-5 (pbk.
: alk. paper)—ISBN (invalid) 978-0-8135-7054-9 (e-book (web pdf))—ISBN
978-0-8135-7361-8 (e-book (epub))
1. Families. 2. Middle class families. 3. Parents of children with disabilities. 4. Children
with disabilities. 5. Children with social disabilities. I. Title
HQ728.F646 2015
306.85—dc23
2014049321

A British Cataloging-in-Publication record for this book is available from the British
Library.

Visit our website: http://rutgerspress.rutgers.edu

Manufactured in the United States of America

To Patricia Lou McGill Woods and
Hayden O'Donnell Woods

CONTENTS

PREFACE

I was drawn to this topic initially not as a parent, but as a sister and a daughter. My brother had struggled for years with substance addiction, and during the times I feared for his life, I worried that I would lose my mother as well. His troubles were her troubles, and, of the two of them, it often seemed like she carried the greater proportion of hardship and sorrow. My interests were also academic and political. Scholarship in the sociology of family had left me highly critical of the child-centered approach to parenthood that has become so taken for granted in our culture. Fashionable models of motherhood, with the mandate to breastfeed and bond and orchestrate children's development, struck me as terribly regressive. In the process of studying a program for gifted children, I also had witnessed first-hand the ramifications of middle-class mothers' school involvement on educational inequality. Why, I wondered, are so many privileged women so deeply invested in motherhood? And what happens when their children, so closely monitored and carefully cultivated, fall short of their expectations?

My son was born several years after I finished collecting data, and by then I was in the process of revising this manuscript for publication. The stories that comprise this book, as well as my own personal experiences, have rendered me more sympathetic to middle-class men and women who find themselves immersed in raising children. I know, now, how the assorted pieces of one's personal life tend to shift position in response to children's gravity. I understand how parental love and responsibility feel elephantine and how most of us are willing to do anything for our children. I am no less critical of popular parenting models and, in particular, of their role in the reproduction of gender inequality. However, I am far more cognizant of the social and historical processes at work on parents' psyches. Children promise us a clear sense of purpose and enduring connection in a society where such things are hard to come by. They are totems, of sorts, in a world with too little magic.

An undergraduate student recently interviewed me for a paper about the process of becoming a parent, and I was struck by how vulnerable I felt during our conversation. It is worth pointing out that this book was possible only because fifty-five people were willing to talk with me, a stranger, in intimate detail about some of the most difficult moments of their lives. Thus, I owe a tremendous debt of gratitude to the parents who were willing to entrust me with their stories.

I am also indebted to the mentors, colleagues, family members, and friends who have supported this work. I was exceedingly fortunate to have been mentored by Lyn Lofland, a first-rate sociologist and steadfast adviser. Lyn trained me in the symbolic interactionist tradition while also encouraging me to think like a generalist. Her careful and critical readings of my work always strengthened the project's momentum, rather than diminished it. Indeed, if there is an art to coaching someone through the grueling work of drafting a first book, Lyn is a master. So is Eviatar Zerubavel, who generously mentored me as I prepared this manuscript for publication. Turning my attention toward the key role of parents' expectations and narratives of self, our conversations sharpened my thinking and strengthened my arguments. I am grateful for his excellent guidance.

I owe thanks to several people who advised me at critical moments in the research and publication process. Laura Grindstaff and Vicki Smith were important sources of direction and support during my time at the University of California, Davis. Anita Ilta Garey provided incisive feedback on my nascent research design and, later, offered much-needed encouragement as I made the transition from graduate student to faculty member. Jennifer Dunn gave me substantive and strategic advice on the book's conceptual framework, and Jerry Lembcke volunteered a number of wise suggestions for how to make the writing more accessible to a public readership. Peter Mickulas's editorial guidance was insightful, supportive, and direct, and I appreciate having had the opportunity to work with the production team at Rutgers University Press.

It is a privilege to work in the Department of Sociology and Anthropology at College of the Holy Cross, where my bright and dedicated colleagues make the halls of Beaven feel like a second home. Renee Beard and Daina Harvey took time out of their summer schedules to read and comment on a full draft of this manuscript, and Jennie Germann-Molz offered feedback as I set out to circulate the prospectus. Susan Rodgers, Sue Crawford Sullivan, and Ed Thompson gave me conceptual and practical advice at different turns. It is hard to imagine having better colleagues.

There were times when pursuing this project required substantial emotional work. Thank goodness for Jill Bakehorn, who helped me keep things in perspective, and for Leila Strickland, who lent a sympathetic ear on more than one occasion. Kim Gordon makes everything easier, particularly when trying to balance the demands of work at home and on campus. I am grateful, too, for the "Vamp" crew. Stephenie Chaudoir, Kendy Hess, Nadine Knight, Jennifer Lieb, and Sarah Webster gave me much-needed respite and camaraderie in the form of network television and take-out food. Finally, I offer gratitude to my friend, colleague, and partner, Ellis Jones, whose faith in my ability to bring this project to fruition has both anchored and animated me. Thank you, Ellis, for always answering "yes," unequivocally and without hesitation, whenever I asked you if this book would see the light of day.

FAMILY TROUBLE

"Your kids are life. You know, if you're the kind of parents that we are, that's what counts. Everything else, you can buy a new car, a new house, who cares? All that stuff. Your kids, that's the one thing, that's the most important thing. So if something is really wrong, significantly wrong... there's no worse trouble in our family than kid-trouble."

—Seth, remembering when his fourteen-year-old daughter ran away from home and was living on the streets

1 • PARENTS IN TROUBLE

Nathan[1] was eleven years old when his parents noticed that something was wrong. He had spent the week at a science camp—it was his first time away from home—and when he came back, he was not himself. His mother, a soft-spoken woman in her early forties, recalled, "Something was off. Something was different . . . [he had] insomnia . . . dark circles under his eyes . . . stomach aches. [He kept] crying in the morning, begging not to go to school. [He was] very panicky." Joan took her son to their pediatrician. Then, when test results indicated that everything was normal, she sought the help of a child psychologist. It took her a while to find a practitioner she trusted, and when she did, the news was not good. "[My son was] having difficulty with cognition and organization of thought. The Rorschach test showed a lot of depression, anxiety, a sense of helplessness . . . he was at risk for suicide." The worst-case scenario, the doctor said, was that Nathan's condition was psychologically degenerative. When Joan asked what that meant, the doctor replied, "Schizophrenia."

Sergio, who is Joan's husband and Nathan's father, remembers how difficult it had been to find a good psychologist in the first place. They had been in and out of so many doctors' offices and received conflicting diagnoses. "We were going to doctors on a weekly basis . . . [one of them] kept going back to attention deficit/hyperactivity disorder, and we knew it wasn't that . . . [then] we had one doctor say he might have a type of cancer in his brain." The thing was, Sergio was not convinced that his son needed a doctor. "He'll grow out of it," he thought. So, even though he dutifully accompanied Joan and Nathan to every appointment, Sergio did not help Joan search for psychologists, and he was not interested in researching his son's symptoms.

Upon hearing the word "schizophrenia," Joan worked around the clock to find a well-respected psychiatrist and effective pharmaceuticals. "Early intervention was key," she said. "I had to keep going until I fixed him." Joan is a mortgage broker, and she was working more than forty hours per week during this period.

It was not long before the stress overwhelmed her. "I was physically and emo-tionally wiped out and drained and fearful of the future. And I couldn't fix my son. . . . [I felt like] it was my *job* to do that and that I would be failing him if I didn't." Eventually, she was diagnosed with fibromyalgia, a condition she attri-butes to the stress associated with Nathan's problems.

Meanwhile, Joan and Sergio were growing apart. Sergio was worried about his son, to be sure. "When the doctor said that the worse case scenario [was] schizo-phrenia and possible suicide, that really freaked me out," he said. "I could just hear my son in his room, talking to the wall or trying to hang himself. [I could imagine myself] waking up in the morning to see him hanging from his ceiling fan." But he rarely expressed these fears to Joan, who became increasingly angry and resentful. "My husband initially would downplay everything. 'Oh, Nathan is doing fine.' When I would express concern . . . I was quickly shut down. Sergio just didn't want to talk about it . . . [he] thought that I was overreacting."

I talked with Joan and Sergio five years after Nathan first developed symp-toms. At that time they still had not received a satisfactory diagnosis, but Nathan's condition was stable, and he was taking medication to prevent a psy-chotic break. Things had gotten better for the three of them, but they were by no means "back to normal." Joan continued to suffer from migraine headaches, neck pain, and fatigue. Sergio was seeing a psychotherapist and, in retrospect, felt awful about having been "in denial" about his son's problems. Joan and Ser-gio had considered separation but were desperately trying to make their mar-riage work. When trying to summarize everything that had happened to them, Joan put it this way: "Pain radiates in the family . . . [when] somebody is ill, to the extent that they can't be the way they were, it just upsets the whole dynamic."

Her comments cut to the heart of the matter. Nathan was no longer himself, no longer the child that she and Sergio had known or imagined him to be. Per-ceiving a change in her son—once a "healthy child," now a "child at risk"—Joan changed too, immersing herself in the research and work related to Nathan's problems. This shift had a profound impact on her physical and psychological health; she, too, was no longer who she used to be. Even Sergio, determined though he was to view his son's condition as a phase, could not avoid the reper-cussions of these changes. Visions of his son's suicide haunted his imagination, and his marital problems led him to a therapist's office where he tried to experi-ence and express emotion in ways that would reconnect him to his family.

This book is about people like Joan and Sergio, middle-class parents whose children have problems. The conditions themselves are quite variable; I inter-viewed the mothers and fathers of children with depression, trichotillomania, attachment disorder, bipolar disorder, autism spectrum disorder, developmen-tal delays, learning disabilities, attention deficit/hyperactivity disorder, drug addiction, alcoholism, truancy, aggression, brain injury, Fragile X syndrome, hyperinsulinism, fetal alcohol syndrome, and cerebral palsy. What ties these parents together is that all identified their children as having "significant problems" and, at one time or another, all had sought the help of experts when trying to remedy those problems. Parts of this book are concerned with mothers' and fathers' varying interpretations of children's conditions and behaviors and the gendered nature of child rearing. Other parts focus on parents' efforts to find effective treatments and to successfully navigate medical and educational bureaucracies. But above all, this book examines how children's problems disrupt middle-class parents' taken-for-granted realities. It captures how, in Joan's words, children's problems "radiate" and spill over into other areas of parents' lives.

Throughout the book, I argue that middle-class parents who identify their children as having significant "problems" experience what I call "family trouble." For Joan and Sergio, "normal" children are a central feature of personal life, and parenthood is a foundation upon which much else depends. Children's problems—or, as I will explain, the collective interpretation of children's conditions and behaviors as problematic—disrupted this foundation, and trouble was the result. My conceptualization of "family trouble" takes up the time-honored sociological tradition of examining how personal troubles are social in nature. I focus primarily on how children's problems resulted in the disruption of micro-social order and the patterns of action and interaction that made up parents' daily lives, but I also situate those patterns in the broad cultural and historical contexts of childrearing and families in the late-Modern West.

This book is not merely about disruption, however. Parents' troubles also reveal the illusory yet powerful nature of "ordinary" children, families, and life trajectories in the late-modern United States. Thus, by focusing on what happens when, from parents' perspectives, "thing go wrong," this book challenges culturally dominant ideas about "normalcy." Privilege, and its role in shaping parents' expectations, is an integral part of that story. Although conditions like Nathan's are not class-specific, their ramifications for parents are. With this book, then, I set out to understand how a relatively affluent group of parents—most of whom are white, heterosexual, college educated, and have steady incomes and homes of their own—made sense of problems that compromised their attainment of what they had imagined to be "the good life."

TROUBLE

Understanding the general concept of "trouble" begins with the premise that life has no inherent meaning. Most of us prefer not to linger over this idea, it seems too serious or too dark, but the notion that human life has no given purpose is an underlying assumption of most, if not all, of the sociological research conducted today. This is because the sociological perspective rests on the notion that reality is socially constructed, and this implies that life's meanings are not inherent but are, instead, generated by human beings. People tend to associate social constructionism with particular schools of thought—ethnomethodology or symbolic interactionism, for example—but in reality, the discipline of sociology has operated under constructionist assumptions since at least the 1930s.[2]

If reality is born of social processes, then it follows that human life has no *inherent* meaning. That is not to say that life is *meaningless*. The need to create meaning, to make sense of life, is just as central to the human condition as the need for food and shelter. This is another foundation of sociological thought. In their study of how the homeless eke out a meaningful existence in the face of dehumanizing conditions, for example, David Snow and Leon Anderson challenged the conventional wisdom that self-worth is a higher-order need than physical comfort.

> All animals are confronted with the challenge of material subsistence, but only humans are saddled with the vexing question of its meaning. We must not only sustain ourselves physically to survive, but we are also impelled to make sense of our mode of subsistence, to place it in some meaningful context, to develop an account of our situation that does not destroy our sense of self-worth. Otherwise, the will to persist falters and interest in tomorrow wanes.[3]

This understanding of the human condition—the notion that meaning resides at the core of human experience and that all meanings are socially constructed—highlights the central importance of society for the individual. It also underscores the fragility of human realities. Society is what shields us from "nothingness."[4] In Peter Berger's words, it "builds a world for us to live in and thus protects us from the chaos that surrounds us on all sides. It provides us with a language and with meanings that make this world believable. And it supplies a steady chorus of voices that confirm our beliefs and still our dormant doubts."[5] At the same time, society emerges from the complex coordination of human conduct and is vulnerable to unexpected events, unanticipated consequences, human error, and willful deviance. From a dramaturgical perspective, people are like "acrobats engaged in perilous balancing acts, holding up between them the swaying structure of the social world."[6] Society, then, is a precarious enterprise. Though it brings meaningful order to human life, it does not once and for all solve the problem of meaning.

The day-to-day work of meaning-making and meaning-maintenance occurs in social interaction. Fundamental assumptions about who we are and how the world operates grow out of, and are continually reinforced, in mundane contexts like homes, workplaces, supermarkets, and sidewalks. The degree to which ontological security, or a person's basic sense of "okay-ness," relies on the smooth operation of everyday interaction is revealed by what happens when routine encounters break down. Nowhere is this demonstrated more clearly than in Harold Garfinkel's classic breaching demonstrations.[7] In one case, Garfinkel asked his students to behave as guests in their own homes. They were polite and impersonal with their family members, using "Mr." and "Mrs." to address their parents, for example, and asking for permission before eating something from the refrigerator. In another case, Garfinkel encouraged students to engage someone in conversation and behave under the assumption that the person had hidden motives and was trying to trick or deceive them. By violating unacknowledged premises of social interaction (relational history in the first case, trust in the second), these demonstrations resulted in bewilderment, anxiety, and anger. The students themselves were deeply uncomfortable, so much so that they found the interactions difficult to sustain and, in some cases, were unable to complete the assignment.

Garfinkel's work illustrates how even small fractures in the structure of microsocial life can threaten an individual's sense of well-being. Even minor interactional failures can lead to anxiety or embarrassment because social order is premised on people adhering to the basic rules of sociability.[8] As human beings, our actions are governed largely by culture, rather than instinct; our knowledge of what to do, and how or when to do it, depends on shared definitions of the situation embedded in larger institutional contexts. When something disrupts the routine flow of interaction and the "rules" no longer seem to apply, we easily lose our bearings.

Given its history in sociology, "trouble" is an appropriate term for the disruption of social order and the subsequent disruption of selves. The classic distinction between "personal troubles" and "public issues" conveys how ostensibly personal problems are linked to larger social and historical circumstances.[9] Research in the "micro-politics of trouble" explores the interpersonal processes by which people recognize, respond to, contest, and construct "problems" in everyday life.[10] Among scholars who conduct conversation analysis, there is a tradition of studying "troubles-talk," or conversations that touch upon problematic events or situations.[11] Finally, gender scholars write about "troubling" gender when a person subverts or confounds the gender binary.[12] Sociologists use the word "trouble" informally, in a way that is consistent with its conventional meaning. "Trouble" is "a problematic departure from the course of ordinary events that warrants special treatment."[13] It begins "when someone experiences dissatisfaction, irritation, upset or discontent with some act or attitude on the part of another."[14] To *make* trouble is to actively disrupt or destabilize.[15] However, these uses of "trouble" also convey something beyond that which is usually implied in casual speech. Sociologists conceive of trouble as a collective phenomenon, a property of interactions, relationships, groups, and institutions. From a socio-logical perspective, trouble manifests *between* people, not just within them. Also, a sociological orientation to trouble is concerned, fundamentally, with the dis-ruption of social order. Trouble is what occurs when the patterns of social life do not unfold as people believe they ought to. In this way, "trouble" is a distinctly sociological concept. In this book, I refine these ideas and deploy the concept of "family trouble" to illuminate parents' experiences of distress.

FAMILY TROUBLE

All interactions are venues for reality maintenance, but not all are of equal importance to the self. Ideologically premised on voluntary commitment, mutual affection, and self-fulfillment, late-modern families are important locales where people form and sustain personal identities.[16] For some people, though certainly not all, family relationships are cherished social spaces where they can be "themselves." Partnership and parenthood also conscript people into roles that organize interaction outside of the family. To be a spouse, mother, father, or child is to occupy a particular place in relationships, and those roles anchor the self to groups, organizations, and institutions.[17] Because families often serve as bedrock for salient personal and social identities, the disruption of family mem-bers' interactions—through separation, illness, or death, for example—can have profound social psychological consequences.[18]

Consider Erving Goffman's "The Insanity of Place," where he describes what it is like for family members living with someone who is manic.[19] The patient's frenetic activity violates the routine order of family life in a number of ways; he or she stops contributing to domestic work, fails to meet even the most mun-dane obligations, squanders the family's money, and, by feverishly forming relationships with anyone who is willing, weakens the boundary between fam-ily members and outsiders. Not only does the manic person violate the family's interaction order, but he or she offers no apologies or excuses for doing so. As Goffman explains, the consequences for family members are more than just pragmatic. In failing to keep his or her "place," the ill person fails to substantiate family members' notions of self and reality.

> In ceasing to know the sick person, [family members] cease to be sure of them-selves. In ceasing to be sure of [the sick person] and themselves, they can even cease to be sure of their way of knowing. A deep bewilderment results. Confirma-tions that everything is predictable and as it should be cease to flow from [the patient's] presentations. The question as to what it is that is going on is not redun-dantly answered at every turn but must be constantly ferreted out anew.[20]

This example of family disruption in the extreme underscores what is at stake in close personal relationships. We depend on the people we love to verify taken-for-granted ideas about ourselves, other people, and the world around us. Only when they remain within the broad margins of who we expect them to be can we rest assured that life is unfolding as it should be.

Defined as an upheaval in family interaction that threatens some salient aspect of the self and results in cognitive and emotional turmoil, "family trouble" captures the dynamic processes of disruption stemming from children's problems. Parents like Joan and Sergio experienced an upheaval in the social structure of everyday life. To varying degrees, their taken-for-granted expectations, daily routines, and personal relationships were organized around rearing "healthy," "normal" children. As a meaningful social anchor, the smooth unfolding of parenthood promised to provide meaning and purpose. Children's problems, then, initiated a chain of disruption that moved through parents' lives in domino-like fashion, culminating in a crisis characterized by uncertainty, loneliness, guilt, grief, and anxiety.

Understanding parents' troubles means that we must take into account the specific social contexts in which they're embedded. Joan and Sergio's troubles cannot be separated from the cultural landscape of parenthood and families in the late-modern United States. As I argue here, the elevated significance of childhood and parenthood makes fertile ground for the type of family trouble these parents experienced.

CHILD-CENTERED LIVES

This book opens with a quote from one of the fathers in this study. "Your kids are life," said Seth, remembering what it was like when his fourteen-year-old daughter ran away. "You know, if you're the kind of parents that we are, that's what counts . . . your kids, that's the one thing, that's the most important thing." For the parents in this study and, indeed, many mothers and fathers across the contemporary West, children are lynchpins around which other important aspects of life revolve. At the most basic level, parenthood anchors a person to a particular set of actions or behaviors. It sets the parameters for what a person *does*. All roles do this to some degree, but parenthood among middle-class people in the United States is a time-intensive enterprise that increases household demands[21] and leaves people with less time for leisure[22] and sleep.[23] Childrearing reorganizes work within and outside of the home, usually in highly gendered ways.[24] It also transforms people's relationships, strengthening some types of connections and weakening others.[25] Finally, parenthood ensnares people's emotions, shaping how they feel and how they are *supposed* to feel. Here, too, childrearing is greedy, constructed as emotionally absorbing, particularly for women.[26] We expect people to love their children, deeply and unconditionally. We also expect parenthood to be emotionally rewarding, despite the much-publicized finding that parents are not as happy as their child-free counterparts.[27] In short, for those who choose to have children in our contemporary context, parenthood is likely to be an organizing centerpiece of personal life. For some, it even can be said to operate as a "master status," or a position that "tends to overpower, in most crucial situations, any other characteristics which might run counter to it."[28]

The weighty importance of parenthood is an interesting phenomenon, given that two demographic shifts in the past fifty years threatened to erode parents' investment in childrearing. The first of these changes was an increase in married mothers' employment. Women's labor force participation rose steadily throughout the 20th century, and some groups of mothers have always worked for pay.[29] However, the paid labor of married mothers increased substantially in the 1970s, and a majority of today's married mothers are employed.[30] The second shift was an increase in single parenting. The divorce rate spiked in the 1970s, and although it plateaued in 1980s, the proportion of children born to unmarried women has continued to rise.[31]

These shifts could have occurred at the expense of "good parenting." We might assume, for example, that because of these trends, today's parents spend less time with their children than parents did in the past or that children are somehow less important to parents than they used to be. However, our best evidence suggests the opposite: today's mothers and fathers are devoted just as strongly, if not more so, to childrearing than their 1960s counterparts were at height of the Baby Boom. Time-diary surveys indicate that today's parents spend more time interacting with their children than parents did in 1965.[32] What's more, the quality of time they spend does not appear to have been compromised. Relative to parents in the 1960s, today's mothers and fathers spend approximately twice as much time on enriching activities such as talking, reading, and playing with their children.[33] Also, despite the competing demands of domestic and paid work, mothers and fathers overwhelmingly report that they enjoy being with their children, even in the relatively mundane contexts of daily caregiving.[34]

Sociologists explain these data in part by looking at countervailing trends that have elevated the place of children in parents' personal lives. Birthrates have been declining for nearly a century, and given the wide availability of contraceptives, people no longer view parenthood as an inevitable part of the life course. The stigma of childlessness has decreased in salience, and for growing segments of the American population, having children is a lifestyle choice.[35] It might be that today's parents spend more time with their children because, relative to previous generations, a greater proportion of them wanted to become parents. At the same time, the symbolic value of children has increased. Unlike previous eras in U.S. history, when children worked and made essential contributions to household economies, today's children spend most of their time in school and are economic liabilities.[36] In the late-modern West, we value children largely for what they symbolize and potentially galvanize within us: innocence, virtue, joy, love, altruism, and deep personal connection. This "pricelessness" encourages deep personal investments in childrearing.

People first imbued children with moral and religious significance in the early 20th century. This process of "sacralization" can be understood, in part, as cultural resistance to the spread of market rationality.[37] Prior to industrialization in the West, there was little separation between personal and public life. Households operated as workplaces, churches, schools, and asylums, and relationships of all kinds were codified by religion, tradition, and personal obligation.[38] As urbanization, the rise of machine production, and the decline of subsistence economies stripped households of their previous functions, people's relationships began to more closely reflect the tenets of modernization: efficiency, competition, impersonal ties, and the pursuit of one's own interests.

In this context, women, children, and "the home" emerged in symbolic opposition to the marketplace and became ideological repositories for unconditional love, moral commitment, and deep personal connection. Some scholars speculate that children's symbolic value has continued to grow precisely because traditional ideas about family life (which never matched lived realities) cannot be sustained in light of late-modern change.[39] In the words of sociologist Allison Pugh,

> As mothers' work lives look more and more like fathers', who but the child is left to sacralize as the vessel of all that is dear about domesticity? As the percentage of single parent households maintains itself at historically high levels, who but the child is left to symbolize family devotion? As community bonds wither, who but the child is left to embody parents' emotional connections?[40]

For the parents featured in this book—especially mothers, as I will illustrate, but fathers too—there is no doubt that children and childrearing are pivotal features of personal life. Children serve as the emotional centers and organizing forces of parents' worlds. It is in this context that children's problems were catalysts for family trouble. Joan and Sergio's story highlights the potential for children's problems to unsettle people's marriages and their role performances as mothers and fathers. However, such problems often reverberated well beyond family life, also disrupting parents' friendships and employment trajectories. To varying degrees, children's maladies resulted in a re-evaluation and reorganization of parents' interpersonal and intrapersonal worlds. Parents struggled not only to make sense of children's problems, but also to make sense of what it meant to be the parent of a "problem child," to envision futures that were quite different from the ones they had planned, and to have a life that no longer seemed "normal."

SELVES, NARRATIVES, AND "NORMAL" LIVES

The upheaval stemming from children's problems played a momentous role in parents' biographies. The disruption of cherished expectations, routines, and relationships transformed parents' selves and, in many cases, led them to feel as though they were no longer "normal." In some parents' minds, family trouble set them apart from an imagined community of middle-class people whose values and goals no longer matched their own. Mothers and fathers often talked about their previous selves, reflecting on the people they had been before their children's problems emerged. Rather than looking back fondly, however, some viewed these past selves as shallow and naïve.

Understanding this dimension of parents' experiences requires a sociological analysis of the self and a critical examination of the role of "normalcy" in self-construction and self-transformation. Self, or the ongoing internal conversation that takes place as we recognize and respond to our own thoughts, feelings, and actions, is best conceptualized as an internalized form of interaction.[41] We tend to think of the self in terms of our separateness from others, but, in actuality, the flow of our internal dialogue continuously shifts as we move across contexts, from one role performance to another, and through the web of relationships and encounters that make up our social milieu. Deeply responsive to the demands of social circumstance, we are, in important respects, different people at different moments in time. This means that our selves are surprisingly fluid, or "open-ended, tentative, exploratory, hypothetical, problematical, devious, changeable, and only partly unified." [42]

Despite this fluidity, we usually experience the self as remaining coherent and consistent over time. In most cases we *desire* personal continuity and actively foster the sense that our personal histories "hang together" or "make sense" in some linear fashion.[43] To the degree that personal instability threatens social order, others demand continuity of us as well;[44] if we are the same from one day to the next, it is easier for people to anticipate our actions and to coordinate their own. The notion of linearity—a life that unfolds in an orderly, undeviating sequence—is particularly characteristic of Western societies.[45] Moreover, we tend to conceive of the "good life" as a moving forward along an "upward-leaning ladder," always progressing, developing, and becoming better over time.[46]

As the parents in this study so clearly demonstrate, actual lives are messy and rarely unfold in a linear or cohesive sequence. Each of us *brings order* to disjointed experiences and events by weaving them into coherent stories about who we are, were, and will be.[47] Continuity, then, is a narrative accomplishment that becomes difficult to maintain when something disrupts the self-stories we've come to take for granted. Prior to the emergence of children's problems (or what came to be seen as problems), parents imagined their own and children's lives as unfolding along a particular trajectory. Children were, parents assumed, headed toward a higher education, marriage, and children of their own. Parents expected to take pride in their performances as mothers and fathers, to someday grow into adult relationships with their children, to become grandparents, and enjoy a retirement free of intensive caregiving. The family troubles described in this book constituted a "turning point," or a critical juncture when a person "takes stock," "re-evaluates," or "revises" her story.[48] Parents' narrative trajectories changed course as they questioned their expectations of children, family life, and the future. Many came to reject their previous assumptions about what constitutes a good life and how much control one can reasonably expect to exert over life's outcomes.

What they experienced was very similar to what sociologists of health and illness call "biographical disruption," or the upending of a person's taken-for-granted worlds and the explanatory frameworks that legitimate them.[49] Parents told new stories as they attempted to make sense of life in the midst of disorder. Just like the wounded storytellers of Arthur Frank's book on illness, parents generated narratives of restitution with plots that hinged on remedying children's problems; narratives of chaos in which parents were consumed by the immediacy of caring for their children and the poignancy of their own grief, guilt, and anxiety; and quest narratives that foregrounded acceptance, resilience, and joy.[50] Parents' experiences illustrate the relevance of biographical disruption beyond studies of illness. What is interesting about this case, though, is that parents themselves did not suffer from a troubling condition; their children did.[51] This highlights how biographical disruption is not primarily an intrapersonal matter, or something that resides within people's minds and bodies. Rather biographical disruption is one component of trouble; it occurs in tandem with the disruption of the micro-social structures in which selves are so deeply embedded.

Indeed, parents revised their narratives of self because children's problems had such a fundamentally disruptive effect on the routines and interactions that sustained their previous stories. Narratives are in all cases embedded in the patterned flow of social life.[52] Stories emerge in interaction with others and are molded, enabled, and constrained by particular audiences. Parents' transformation into mothers and fathers whose children "have problems" grew out of their relationships to one another, their encounters with medical professionals and schoolteachers, and their interactions with family members, friends, acquaintances, and even strangers. Situated more broadly within a culture of risk and hyper-vigilance,[53] an ideology of intensive motherhood and pervasive mother-blame,[54] and the widespread pathologization of difference,[55] these interactions fostered parents' redefinitions of their children and themselves.

Beneath multiple layers of disruption and self-change, parents grappled with the sense that they were no longer "normal." But what is normal? The concept is such a pivotal, taken-for-granted feature of how we think about human variation that we rarely question its meaning. However, the whole notion that some characteristics are "regular," "average," or "standard" while others are "irregular," "aberrant," or "deviant" is a social construct that did not emerge in Western cultures until the mid-19th century. Prior to this period, there were literary and artistic representations of the "ideal," but such forms were tied to the divine and, by definition, not humanly attainable.[56] Only with the emergence of statistics and the bell-shaped curve did the idea of "normalcy" take root in the collective imagination.[57] What is interesting, though, is that "the norm"—ostensibly meant to describe what is "typical"—became the ideal. In everyday speech, commonly held ideas about "normal people" with "normal families" do not reflect a statistical middle. Instead, "normal" is a moral and political category that serves to elevate some families and delegitimize others.[58] That we see "normal" as an enviable position is, in fact, part of its legacy as a statistical construct; most early statisticians were eugenicists who hoped to eliminate "undesirable" deviation and improve the human race.[59]

"Normal," then, does not refer to "what is" but is a set of ideas about what "should be." Its content and boundaries are hazy, largely imperceptible until juxtaposed with the "not normal." In terms of the self, it is precisely during periods of disruption and transformation that "normal" comes into focus and begins to loom large. The parents I interviewed expected to have "normal" children but said they had been unaware of and unable to articulate the content of these expectations until they came to view their children as "having problems." Prior to this turning point, they had not necessarily used the framework of "normal" to define themselves or their families, but this designation became an important way of talking about their previous selves and how children's problems had changed them. In light of their families' troubles, many parents came to see certain friends and acquaintances as belonging to a group of "normal," middle-class people with whom they now had little in common. Some men and women expressed gratitude for this dis-identification and believed that they were better, more compassionate people for having suffered. In this way, "normalcy" was a foil, serving as a narrative backdrop against which parents constructed new selves.

Scholars in critical disability studies have critiqued the concept of biographical disruption precisely because "normalcy" is a constructed, deeply political category. If not deployed carefully, the framework of disruption reifies or essentializes distinctions between health and illness, ability and disability, or typical and atypical. It can give the impression that certain conditions or behaviors are inherently problematic or inevitably disruptive. As critical scholars rightly point out, disability and illness are not *in the body*.[60] Rather, these are sets of meanings that people attach to certain types of physical and intellectual difference. In this view, illness and disability serve as forms of social oppression that deny full personhood and block equal participation in social life.[61] The framework of disruption, some argue, unwittingly endorses the pathologization of difference and takes for granted meanings that are, in actuality, socially constructed.[62]

On one hand, this critique is well-founded and closely aligns with the constructionist orientation I take in this book. I argue that there is nothing inevitable about parents' troubles, and I analyze how their experiences of disruption emerged not from children's conditions and behaviors, per se, but from the micro-political processes of interpreting those conditions and behaviors. I also explore the dynamics of social exclusion that punctuated parents' experiences, paying close attention to the moral assumptions embedded in conceptions of what is "normal." On the other hand, the parents I interviewed viewed their children's conditions and behaviors as *problems* and understood their own experiences in terms of disruption. They talked about unfulfilled expectations and loss and used words like "devastation" and "trauma." Their experiences are not universal, and, as I discuss in Appendix A, I designed this study in ways that invited stories of disruption. Nonetheless, "trouble" is a fitting conceptual framework because it captures disruption *as parents experienced it.*

Critically analyzing family trouble from the constructionist perspective while also doing justice to parents' suffering presents a dilemma of language. Children's "problems" are the products of micro-political processes, yes, but they are simultaneously real and obdurate features of parents' lives. Problems of every sort are socially constructed, but, to paraphrase W. I. Thomas's famous dictum, if people define situations as real, they are real in their consequences.[63] What is the best way to write about children's problems, then? Should I use quotation marks to remind the reader that "the problems" are not inherent to children's conditions or behaviors but emerged, instead, from social interaction and collective interpretation? Or should I allow such words as "normal," "problems," and "troubles" to remain unquoted, given the stubborn, factual quality of their operation in these parents' everyday worlds? Insofar as social conditions are both processes and structures, neither of these orientations is inaccurate. Thus, my language vacillates throughout the book. When my aim is to examine the processes by which "problems" are constructed or to highlight the illusory nature of "normalcy," I use quotation marks. However, when my aim is to illuminate the micro-social consequences of those problems or to provide the readers with an understanding of what parents' troubles *felt* like, I leave the words unquoted. The latter is also a small measure of respect for the participants in this study, who experienced their children's problems as social facts that tore through their lives with independent force.

In the end, my analysis of family trouble conveys an overarching sociological lesson about what is, or what might *seem*, "normal." At one time or another, all of us possess a stigmatizing characteristic that violates dominant cultural ideas about what is "ordinary," "acceptable," "moral," or "worthy."[64] Because no child, family, or life course can altogether adhere to what medical anthropologist Gay Becker calls "normalizing ideologies,"[65] most of us will at some point feel a sense of loss, disorientation, or difference because something in our personal lives seems to have "gone wrong." Though we usually think of disruption as some kind of *deviation* from what is typical, it is part of the human condition.[66] By bringing dominant cultural ideals about children, families, and "the good life" into clear view—and by highlighting the relatively narrow and class-specific nature of those ideals—the sociological perspective offers a clear message to anyone in the throes of family trouble: you are in good company, and you are not as different as you might feel.

VARIATION, HOMOGENEITY, AND SPEAKING GENERALLY

The parents in this book identified their children as having problems of various sorts that ranged from mild to severe. I talked with biological parents, as well as adoptive parents. Some had been grappling with their children's problems for years and others had only recently come to believe that something was wrong. Is it reasonable, or even possible, to bracket such broad variation and say something meaningful about these parents as a group?

When I set out to collect data, I deliberately welcomed disparate cases in order to identify the patterns that transcended them. Here I follow in the tradition of what Eviatar Zerubavel calls "social pattern analysis," where the researcher's goal is to "uncover generic patterns invisible to anyone interested only in the specific."[67] Unlike the ethnographer or historian who seeks to examine, describe, or analyze one particular context, this approach allows the analyst to speak generally about patterns that are observable *across* contexts. This mode of inquiry relies on "multi-contextual evidence" drawn from different circumstances, cultures, or historical periods.[68] The data can vary even in terms of scale, moving across the micro–macro divide, but in all cases the researcher's comparisons are meant to identify common patterns. This requires a well-honed analytical focus that permits the researcher to disregard the particular features of each case in order to engage in abstraction and conceptualization.

Social pattern analysis has a long, though often unrecognized, history in sociology.[69] Erving Goffman deployed it, premising the concept of stigma not on the experiences of one disparaged group, for example, but on the experiences of many.[70] Eviatar Zerubavel uses it in his book *Hidden Rhythms*, drawing examples from sources as variable as the Talmud and *Robinson Crusoe*, to demonstrate the powerful, organizing force of sociotemporality.[71] Diane Vaughan employs a similar approach in her study of separation and divorce, interviewing people who had been married for decades, as well as those who had been living with a partner for only a few years.[72] Some of the relationships Vaughan studied were still "in transition" at the time of the interview, while others had ended years ago. Helen Rose Fuchs Ebaugh also takes this methodological orientation in *Becoming an Ex*, collecting stories from ex-doctors, widows, ex-nuns, divorcees, transsexuals, retirees, and mothers without custody, among others.[73] These scholars recognize but bracket variation in order to focus on what is common among their selected cases: generic processes related to stigma, time, uncoupling, and role exit, respectively. Each work then yields a conceptual framework that sensitizes scholars to possibilities in other empirical contexts.[74] This book follows the same logic. Although parents' stories are variable along a number of dimensions, I focus on the remarkably similar patterns of disruption that stemmed from having a child with problems.

Speaking generally does not preclude taking account of difference. Invisible and ill-defined problems posed special challenges for the mothers of school-aged children, for example, because they required high levels of advocacy and rendered women more susceptible to mother-blame. In contrast, people attributed some degree of agency and culpability to teenaged children with substance abuse problems; this curtailed parents' own sense of responsibility, but also made the grief of parents' estrangement from their children difficult to bear. When variations such as problem type or children's ages seemed to shape how people experienced or made sense of disruption, I explore those patterns.

In any case, all of the parents I interviewed told their stories from the beginning, when they first began to suspect that something might be wrong. Each described what things had been like at their worst, and, for those who believed they were "on the other side," time had not altogether dulled the emotional salience of their memories. Indeed, the fear that Sergio experienced when he imagined his son talking to himself or committing suicide is no less real for having been experienced five years prior to our interview. In this way, parents' stories are comparable, even though they unfold along different timelines.

Although children's problems were diverse, the sample is somewhat uniform in other respects. As I mentioned before, this book is, quite intentionally, a study of middle-class parents. Also, with few exceptions, the participants are Caucasian and heterosexual. Because mainstream American culture privileges white, middle-class, heterosexual experience, it is temping to view this group as "the standard" or "norm." For a number of reasons, some of which I have already touched upon, to do so would be a mistake. I chose to study this group of parents, not because they are representative, but because previous research suggests they are anomalous. Although the rise of child-centered parenting is a far-reaching cultural change, parenthood is a class-specific and status-enhancing project. Affluent men and women are more likely to postpone childbearing until they have achieved other culturally-defined goals and believe they are ready to devote generous amounts of time and energy to parenthood.[75] Data illustrate that the average amount of time that people spend with their children increases with income and education.[76] Moreover, status anxiety encourages middle-class parents to orchestrate educational and extracurricular activities in hopes that their children will garner the skills necessary to become successful, middle-class adults.[77] This "concerted cultivation" approach requires high levels of personal investment, potentially making children's problems all the more disruptive.

Constructions of "normality," "disability," and "deviance" are not universal either, and the behaviors or conditions that white, middle-class, heterosexual parents deem to be "problematic" may not be deemed so in other contexts.[78] There is little doubt that race informs people's interpretations and experiences of children's "problems." As I discuss in Chapter 6, the parents in this study associated certain kinds of "problems"—such as underachievement, substance abuse, truancy, and fighting—with poor and working-class non-whites, and this led them to feel as though children's differences had caused them to lose status. In sum, the parents in this study occupy a particularly privileged social location, and their experiences—however variable—cannot be taken to represent other groups.

OVERVIEW

For most parents, trouble emerged slowly as they came to view their children as having "significant problems." Pervasive uncertainty accompanied the growing concern that something was awry. Perceiving their children as having departed from the "norm," parents wondered what was wrong, how it could be fixed, and what it would mean for the future. They found no easy answers. To complicate matters, mothers, fathers, family members, teachers, and doctors often disagreed about the existence, nature, and future repercussions of children's "problems." In Chapter 2, I examine the dynamics of "problem" construction, paying special attention to parents' efforts to develop working consensus in the midst of disagreement and ambiguity.

In Chapters 3 and 4, I explore the disruption of parents' daily lives on two, interrelated fronts: routines and relationships. Children's problems required so much attention and care that they usually became the center of family life and left mothers, especially, with less time and energy to meet other obligations, take care of themselves, or simply enjoy life. The busyness of trying to identify and treat children's problems exhausted parents, while also unsettling their relationships with one another, friends, and other family members. Stigma and ongoing disagreements about children's "problems" were additional sources of relationship disruption and compounded parents' feelings of isolation and otherness. More than just a result of children's problems, the disruption of parents' routines and relationships further contributed to their view that children had significant "problems."

I explore the emotional ramifications of children's problems in Chapters 5. Though few had given it much thought, parents had harbored a set of very particular, class-specific assumptions about their children's life trajectories. Losing the "normal" child who hits the key benchmarks of a "well-lived life" was a profound loss for the men and women in this study, not only because "ordinary children" were key features in their own biographical narratives, but also because of the ostensibly sacred nature of the parent–child bond in our contemporary social context. Most parents were also plagued by anxiety, self-doubt, and guilt, stemming either from the notion that they may have caused children's problems or from the idea that they may have not done enough to ameliorate them. In the wake of such intrapersonal turmoil, many parents said that they had been depressed, and approximately one-third had sought the help of professional therapists. Suffering further disrupted parents' relationships and routines, thereby contributing to the escalation of their troubles.

In Chapter 6, I explore the disruption of parents' selves and consider how family trouble led participants to revise their biographical narratives. In light of children's problems, parents could not sustain the stories they once told about themselves as mothers and fathers, as professionals, and as people in general. As they revised their narratives, they came to dis-identify from the imagined middle-class "mainstream" and separate themselves from the ostensibly "normal" parents who seemed to populate their communities. By refining the concept of anomie to capture parents' disconnection from the worlds they identified with, I reflect on the social nature of parents' suffering. Here I also examine parents' attempts to re-anchor themselves in social space and tell new stories that aligned them with parents in similar situations. Despite the deeply painful experiences associated with children's problems, many parents said that they were grateful for having suffered. The dismantling and rebuilding of taken-for-granted assumptions about themselves, their families, and "the good life" appeared to provide some with more meaningful priorities and greater compassion for others. However, not all parents told stories of positive transformation. The best that some parents could say is that they were trying their best to "make do."

I conclude by considering the relevance of parents' experiences to other studies of family and family-related upheaval. As I explain, late-modern Western families are less rigid than their early-modern counterparts, but the expectation of deep personal investment in family life is, somewhat conversely, greater than ever before. Because families are, for some, a profound source of meaning, purpose, and personal connection, events such as illness, separation or divorce, and death can shake a person's ontological security. The concept of "family trouble," I suggest, allows us to think about generic processes of family-related disruption that stem from seemingly disparate events.

2 • CONSTRUCTING TROUBLE, LOSING CERTAINTY

I arrived at Jen and Carl's house at eight o'clock, just as Carl was pulling into the driveway with the takeout that he and Jen had ordered for dinner. They said they preferred to eat after the interview. With four children, they rarely spent time alone and looked forward to the prospect of sharing a late meal after everyone had gone to bed. Jen and Carl's daughters—ages eight and thirteen—are adopted, and both have special needs. I began our conversation by asking them about their decision to adopt and how they came to discover that their first daughter, Becca, might have problems requiring professional care. They explained that they had been in their early twenties when they decided to have children. An earlier pregnancy had ended in a miscarriage, and Jen was only twenty-four weeks pregnant with a second child when she went into pre-term labor. Doctors performed an emergency caesarean section, but they were unable to save the baby. They told Carl and Jen that future pregnancies would be risky, requiring extended bed rest. The couple, utterly traumatized by this experience, started researching adoption possibilities.

After deciding that they would adopt locally, they signed up to become foster parents and met Becca a mere thirty days after receiving the county's approval to provide care. Just twenty-months old, Becca was living in a foster home that Jen described as "pretty awful," where one family was "warehousing" six young children. Carl was hesitant about adoption, but Jen knew right away that Becca was the one. When I asked the couple if they knew Becca was going to have problems, Jen replied, "Uh-huh, it was very clear to me . . . and I wasn't believed. I think that's because she had attachment issues, and it was not understood back then. . . . I kept asking social workers, 'She's aggressive in a way that doesn't fit. . . .' She didn't feel pain at first. She had really a lot of trouble sleeping." Carl added,

"There was a lot of physical stuff. They only fed her blended foods in this [foster] home. . . . She couldn't swallow very well. She gagged on [solid food]."

Because Becca had been exposed to drugs in utero and neglected in her previous foster home, it was difficult for Jen and Carl to determine the source of these conditions and behaviors. Would they disappear once Becca was appropriately cared for? Carl and Jen wondered if their daughter would have ongoing problems because of her background, but friends and family members were skeptical. Jen commented, "It was very hard to discern what was what, and a lot of people said, 'Oh, you're just being an intense first-time mom.'"

As Becca grew older, however, other behaviors began to manifest. Jen and Carl described their daughter's problems in the following terms:

JEN: [Becca] is very greedy. She's very afraid of losing something or not having enough of something. She never hoarded food, but the minute we'd sit down at that table she would look and make sure it goes to her first. She still does that . . . she has trouble socially. I don't think she really made a good friend until fifth-grade. It took a long time. . . . She raged too. She had a lot of rages . . . and she'd rip everything off her walls.

CARL: She's really had a lot of fears . . . and she still does. . . . Little things can just put her up over the edge to where she's just absolutely terrified. . . . We had an incident where somebody broke the side window of our car and stole [Jen's] purse out of it. . . . And we didn't see any of this, we just came and the window was broken, her purse was gone, and [Becca] . . . was scared to death. . . . She just really lost it and started screaming. . . . So she has issues with that kind of thing.

Jen and Carl sought expert help as a matter of course. They saw numerous doctors over the course of a few years, but it was not until Jen read about attachment disorders that they sought the help of a specialist and received a diagnosis. Now thirteen years old, Becca is thought to have an attachment disorder and takes the anti-depressant medication Paxil.

As Jen and Carl's story illustrates, parents' troubles usually emerged slowly over the course of weeks, months, and years as they came to view their children as having significant "problems." Uncertainty was a heavy burden during these prolonged periods. Even when children had clear physical conditions, such as seizures, the causes and future repercussions of these "symptoms" were not necessarily discernible at the outset. Many of the parents I interviewed were initially unsure about whether or not their children even *had* "problems." As the parent of any young child can attest, tantrums are commonplace. Toddlers acquire language and develop motor skills at varying rates. We expect teenagers to be moody, and for a large proportion of them to drink alcohol or use drugs. Even "normal" children sometimes get poor grades or have a difficult time making friends. How, then, did parents distinguish between the everyday "problems" of "normal children" and the serious, underlying "problems" experienced by "problem children"? This is the question I set out to address in this chapter.

My analysis focuses on the micro-social dynamics of "problem" construction, or what Robert Emerson and Sheldon Messinger call the "micro-politics of trouble."[1] I focus in particular on how parents reached a working consensus given the indeterminate and often contentious nature of children's "problems." Biomedical accounts of difference, social comparisons, and the validation of friends or family members encouraged parents to seek expert intervention. These processes culminated in key turning points as parents came to view their children's conditions and behaviors as "seriously problematic," rather than as "normal," "insignificant," or "temporary." Mothers usually shepherded the interpretive process, though they did so in response to the ever-present threat of mother-blame. I argue that parents' on-the-ground, definitional work was embedded in three broad and interrelated social contexts: a culture of risk that encourages attunement to potential "problems,"[2] an ideology of intensive motherhood that holds women responsible and culpable for children's well-being,[3] and the widespread pathologization and medicalization of childhood.[4] These three features of late-modern American life, I argue, are the larger backdrop against which parents' troubles emerged.

EARLY SUSPICIONS

Concern that something might be wrong with one's child is not an experience limited to parents whose children have "serious problems." Worry and self-doubt are defining features of middle-class parenthood in the contemporary United States.[5] The readiness with which the parents in this study came to view their children's conditions and behaviors as requiring expert intervention must be understood, at least in part, as emerging from a culture of risk that encouraged them to be vigilantly aware of potential "problems."[6] Gone are the days when extended kin and large numbers of siblings share the tasks of childrearing. The nuclear family model finds parents like the ones in this study in relative seclusion with their children, without the accumulated wisdom and helpful hands of grandmothers, aunts, or cousins.[7] Armed with few governing traditions and faced with a proliferation of knowledge claims about children's health and development, these parents (and mothers, in particular, as I will discuss) were already anxious to make sure that their children were okay.

Unlike other worried parents, though, the mothers and fathers in this study eventually determined that their children needed serious help. They reached this conclusion quickly when their children exhibited certain physical conditions, such as seizures. However, many of the conditions and behaviors that initially caused concern—underachievement in school or sports, disobedience, inappropriate presentations of self, not developing or behaving according to one's age, and mild physical ailments like insomnia or stomach aches—contained multiple interpretive possibilities and could be easily seen as the "ordinary problems" of "normal" children. Thus, many parents' troubles began with nebulous feelings of uneasiness and uncertainty. Carol's son was thirteen years old at the time of our interview and was diagnosed with Asperger's syndrome when he was four. Carol recalled how awareness of her son's differences dawned slowly during the first few years of his life.

> Around a year old, we began to notice that he was very hypersensitive to sound, like [the] vacuum cleaner. He was a very intense baby. . . . [We] put him in a toddler class when he was about two. [He] didn't want anything to do with the other kids, absolutely nothing. Cried, fussed, tended to be a very picky eater. Terrified of water splashing on him. . . . I began to start thinking, This is not normal. This is not right.

Carol's comments hint at how children's early "symptoms" seemed like a haphazard assortment of dots. It was only later that labels and diagnoses allowed parents to make connections between them. Steve's seventeen-year-old daughter Margo was in an out-of-state, residential treatment program for cocaine addiction at the time of our interview. He and his wife had felt as though something had been the matter for months, but they could not put a finger on it. Margo had been a competitive water polo player for years but suddenly wanted off the team. Steve explained,

> We would have these discussions, "Margo, what is going on? What's behind [this]? . . . You love this for twenty years, and now all the sudden you hate this. And you hate [your coach] and you hate [your teammates], and everything's eff this and eff that? Margo, what's going on?" . . . We had those . . . discussions, and yeah they were confrontational to some degree . . . . And in the back [of our minds] we never made that link. . . . We just thought it was behavioral.

In an attempt to put words to the emerging sense that something was "wrong," many parents first framed worrisome conditions and behaviors as developmental phases, harmless acts of rebellion, or quirky aspects of their children's personalities. Paula's son was eight years old at the time of our interview but was diagnosed with attention deficit/hyperactivity disorder when he was five. A few years prior to her son's ADHD diagnosis, Paula noticed his strange and inappropriate behavior but did not give it much thought.

I first noticed with the food. He would always eat really rapidly, whatever it was. And then when he would play, he never really played appropriately with toys. He'd either break them, throw them, he would tie 'em in knots. . . . And so I just thought, "Well, that's just his way in the world." I never really thought beyond it. Then when he was three, he was aggressive toward his younger sister. . . . He'd push her down out of the blue. So I would see impulsive behavior, but once again I just kind of dismissed it.

Parents whose children were later diagnosed with an autism spectrum disorder or developmental delay tried to assure themselves that their children were just "late talkers" or "late bloomers." "Boys will be boys" was a common way to make sense of sons' disobedience,[8] and "laziness" explained the underachievement of sons and daughters alike.

In the case of all eventual "problems," the perception that something is "wrong" is often vague, at least at the onset.[9] Problems—or, more accurately, the conditions and behaviors that come to be seen as "problems"—are essentially indeterminate because, regardless of their etiologies, their meanings emerge from social interaction. As I explained in the previous chapter, to assert that children's problems are socially constructed is not to claim that they are not real. On the contrary, "problems" become real when people identify and respond to them as such. Even obdurate physical realities require interpretation in order to have meaningful social consequences. An unknown disease is analogous to "the tree falling in the forest with no ear to hear."[10] Parents' initial attempts to define the situation as "unproblematic"—or, at the very least, nothing *seriously* troublesome—usually prevailed until a critical mass of other people echoed parents' feelings of unease, as I later discuss. In nearly all cases, though, mothers played the lead role in redefining their situations as "troublesome."

MOTHERS AND THE MICRO-POLITICS OF TROUBLE

Mothers in the contemporary West traverse difficult cultural terrain. In her book *The Cultural Contradictions of Motherhood*, Sharon Hays finds that an ideology of intensive mothering encourages women to "expend a tremendous amount of time, energy, and money in raising their children."[11] Premised on the assumption that mothers alone can meet children's increasingly complex needs, this ideology holds women responsible for cultivating children's physical, social, and emotional development. People have long thought mothers culpable for children's successes and failures.[12] However, an obsession with risk has made the task of keeping children healthy and happy seem especially gargantuan. Today, "good mothering" pivots on women's ability to recognize and manage risk.[13] Children's "problems," in turn, cast suspicion on mothers' mastery over myriad, potentially harmful contingencies.

As primary caregivers highly attuned to risk—and as the primary targets of potential blame—it was nearly always mothers who first defined children's conditions and behaviors as "problematic." Fathers were more likely to persist in the interpretation that children's conditions and behaviors were "normal," "temporary," or "insignificant."[14] Sarah and Matt, for example, each had two children when they met ten years ago, and their blended family is tightly-knit. Christopher, who is Matt's seventeen-year-old biological son, has had substance abuse "problems" for two years. When I interviewed this couple together, they said that until school officials found Christopher in possession of drugs, Matt was reluctant to believe there was any cause for concern. He said, "The problem before then was not knowing exactly what he was doing, [and] maybe still on my part going, 'Well . . . boys will be boys . . . he may need to experience something . . . because he's not going to learn any way else.'" In contrast, Sarah had been concerned about Christopher's behavior long before this incident, and she had tried to convince Matt that they should intervene. She said,

> I've been more suspicious. I've seen evidence. I'm more detail-oriented anyway, but I notice and I say to [Matt], "Oh, he seemed high," or, "What's he doing right now? When's he coming back?" . . . There were some months or years where I think it was more difficult because we didn't know really what was going on. We still don't know exactly what's going on with [him], but at least [now] we're more on the same page . . . we understand that there's a drug issue here.

Clearly, Sarah was more attuned than Matt to the possibility of serious "problems." The vigilance she exercised as she gathered "evidence" of her stepson's drug use is precisely the kind of anxious reflexivity that characterizes mothers' pervasive efforts to manage risk.

Sarah and Matt's conflicting interpretations of the situation had been a source of marital tension, a dynamic that was common across problem type. For a long time, Matt had dismissed Sarah's concerns, as illustrated in this brief exchange.

MATT: I think I just thought that you were really suspicious.
SARAH: That I was suspicious?
MATT: Yeah, and then you were right.

Similarly, Martha's thirteen-year-old daughter had struggled in school since kindergarten, and Martha was convinced that her daughter must have a learning disability. Her husband disagreed. Martha recalled,

One of the hardest things was my husband's denial. . . . He was in denial. Kind of the guy-macho-thing, "There's nothing wrong with my kid. . . . We can remedy this. We just have to work harder. She doesn't have a problem. What's this dyslexia thing? That's crazy, that's ridiculous. No, no," simply, "No."

Kathy, whose six-year-old son was diagnosed with cerebral palsy before his first birthday, made similar comments: "[My husband] didn't understand. . . . He's like, 'What's the big deal? That's just [our son]. It's just [our son]. It's no big deal.' You know, it's like, 'No, it's not just [our son] . . . there's more to it than just that.'" Women often used the word "denial" to describe fathers' states of mind. Indeed, a number of mothers associated denial with masculinity and said that fathers were, by nature, slow to acknowledge children's "problems." Carol, whose thirteen-year-old son was diagnosed with Asperger's Syndrome when he was four, said,

[My husband is] a very quiet man. And I think we find [that is true of] most of the men in my support group [for parents whose children have autism]. . . . They tend to be in a lot of denial.

Responses thought to indicate "denial" are common when the meanings of an illness are ambiguous.[15] From a constructionist perspective, fathers' reluctance to frame their children's conditions or behaviors as indicative of "serious problems" was an alternative, but no less valid, definition of the situation.

Fathers were not the only ones who questioned the legitimacy of what mothers viewed as children's emerging "problems." Friends and family members sometimes discounted women as paranoid. Kathy, quoted earlier, recalled that after she voiced concerns about her son's development, "Everyone was telling me, 'Oh you're just paranoid, knock it off. He's fine.'" People also intimated that women are naturally prone to worrying about their children, such as when Jen's friends suggested that she was just being an "intense first-time mom." Stereotypes about the anxious and emotional nature of mothers—and women more generally—probably nurtured people's tendencies to reject mothers' early suspicions.

When family members, friends, or educational professionals did view children's conditions or behaviors as "problematic," they sometimes viewed those emerging "problems" as seated in the relationship between the parent (usually the mother) and the child, rather than within the child's body or mind. Carol said that the teachers at her son's school kept implying that she and her husband were doing something wrong.

CAROL: [The teachers were] asking me things like, "[Mrs. Mathews], do you and your husband"—because [our son's] got such bizarre behavior—"Do you all take drugs? Do you all beat each other?"

ARA: You had people ask you that?

CAROL: Oh yes. *Oh* yes . . . they kept thinking, "Well, he's OCD, and certainly you all must be doing something to encourage this bizarre behavior."

In a few cases, mother-blame was at the center of men's and women's disagreements about children's "problems" too. Megan and Craig, for example, divorced when their daughter was in third-grade. Now sixteen, Kaitlyn takes medication for emotional "problems" and was recently taken to the hospital when she took an overdose of two over-the-counter medications. Megan recalled when she first started to suspect her daughter might suffer from depression.

[Kaitlyn] was starting to act . . . moderately depressed. And she was doing some weird stuff. She was complaining about the kids at school staring at her . . . "nobody liked her" and "they were staring at her" and she started wearing dark glasses a lot, and she'd never really worn sunglasses before. . . . She starts wearing a big, thick, wool, black, long coat. . . . You know, weird stuff. I knew something was going on. And [her] dad was denying it.

Craig, who I interviewed at a separate time, disagreed with Megan's assessment of their daughter's behavior. He believed that Megan's decision to seek professional help was part of an ongoing custody dispute. He said,

[Our daughter was] a perfectly happy kid who is undeniably very intelligent. . . . Now she's on umpteen different drugs—anti-depressants, mood stabilizers, blah blah, all this stuff—that a perfectly normal kid should never have had to go on. [But Megan] had a very vested interest in having [our daughter] declared depressed. . . . She was shopping around to different psychologists to try to get her a diagnosis of mental illness so that she could claim that [our daughter] shouldn't be living with me.

Most mothers eventually convinced fathers of their definition of the situation by claiming to have a better understanding of children and their conduct. As I discuss in the next chapter, many threw themselves into research pertaining to children's "problems," using information garnered from libraries, the Internet, and support groups to persuade their spouses that children had particular kinds of "problems." Martha, for example, kept showing her husband excerpts from the books she had been reading in order to convince him that their daughter, thirteen at the time of our interview, suffered from a learning disability. She said, "I would come in with my new book, my new self-help, kid-has-a-problem book, and say, 'Well, check out this paragraph. Doesn't this sound like her? . . . read this part.'" Because they were usually children's primary caregivers, some women won definitional victories by default. Claire, whose nine-year-old son was diagnosed with autism when he was three, explained,

> I was doing the research. See, [my husband] owns a business in [another city], he only lives here half-time. And at that point, he was only here three days a week. So I was the one who was here. And I just felt like I was more equipped to make the decisions. And so I always lay out the information to him, but he always says, "Yeah, you're right." . . . It's just that I know how to research. He doesn't as much. . . . I teach so I'm into education, and from the very beginning . . . I've always been incredibly involved, as a volunteer, organizer, everything.

Thus, children's "problems" and parents' woes emerged as all troubles emerge: from micro-political processes. Parents had vested interests in the interpretive struggle over children's situations, and they vied for shared understandings that aligned with their own perspectives. Mothers and fathers alike wanted to do what was best for their children. Nonetheless, intensive motherhood and a heightened attention to risk facilitated women's greater readiness to define their children as having "significant problems." A heavy sense of responsibility and the ever-present threat of mother-blame placed women in the defensive position of accounting for children's conduct. Identifying and defining "the problem" suggested particular courses of treatment and, as I explain in Chapter 4, often seated "the problem" firmly within the child, rather than between mother and child. Nonetheless, the decision to seek psychological or medical evaluation was informed by more than just a desire to help children, manage risk, or evade blame, as I discuss next.

BIOMEDICAL ACCOUNTS OF DIFFERENCE

Claire is the mother of a nine-year-old boy diagnosed with autism. At the age of three, her son was often unresponsive and had not acquired much language. Claire said that she did not hesitate to begin "pushing" her son's doctor for an explanation. "I said [to his pediatrician], 'He doesn't respond. Watch!' . . . so [the doctor] said to [my son], 'Where's the table?' . . . I told him, 'If he even glanced at the table I would fall out of my chair. . . . Does he have a learning disability? Does he have a language disorder? What's happening?'"

As this example illustrates, some mothers simply assumed that their children's "problematic" conduct stemmed from biomedical conditions requiring expert intervention. The widespread problematization and medicalization of childhood no doubt encouraged this interpretive orientation. The social construct of childhood emerged in the 19th century and was, from the very beginning, enmeshed with concerns about children's physical, emotional, and psychological development.[16] It is not simply that children's "problems" are medicalized in the late-modern West; children and childhood themselves are objects of elaborate medical surveillance and control. Nonetheless, my own data suggest that women were more or less apt to seek medical accounts, depending on their personal histories. Eleven mothers had studied or worked in the areas of childcare, education, nursing, or mental health. These educational and professional backgrounds alerted them to the possibility of biomedical "problems" and/or made them particularly likely to see children's conditions and behaviors in biomedical terms. For example, Kathy, whose six-year-old son was diagnosed with cerebral palsy before his first birthday, said that she knew the signs of developmental disabilities because of her job.

> [Let me tell you] a little bit about my background: I had been working with special-needs children for ten years prior to having [my son]. So I kind of noticed little things. His eyes were bouncing, his head would bounce, some movements that weren't normal. . . . And I was like, "There's just something not right."

Jessica, a child psychologist whose six-year-old son had been having social and behavioral "problems" since he was four, might have maintained that her son was simply an "intense" child. Instead, she readily adopted the clinical language of her discipline and framed his behavior in terms of pathology: "it's been a struggle to figure out what exactly it is because he doesn't really fit into any true category. He's got a little flavor of bipolar, he's got a flavor of autism, um, but doesn't meet any of the diagnostic criteria for that, for those um . . . I think he has a non-verbal learning disability. He has a really, uh, large spread between his verbal and performance IQ." In several cases, family members, friends, or parents themselves had suffered from maladies similar to those displayed by their children. If mothers were in the practice of using medical accounts to explain comparable "symptoms," they were likely to use them again when making sense of their children's conditions and behaviors. Cynthia's eighteen-year-old daughter has taken medication for depression since she was in the ninth grade. As Cynthia explained,

> [My daughter] said, "I'm just really depressed, and I can't shake it." And I said, "Okay." Went over, made an appointment [with the doctor], came back and said, "Are you suicidal?" And she said, "No." And she said that, "I just don't feel like myself." And I said, "Fine." And so she went and talked to our family doctor, and she was put on an anti-depressant, which she is still on. . . . I suffer from

depression . . . and my brother committed suicide in his late twenties, and so I just don't take it lightly.

In sum, while medicalization might have encouraged most parents to pathologize aspects of their children's development, mothers' personal histories informed their willingness to seek expert advice.

SOCIAL COMPARISONS

Parents also made specific social comparisons that led them to believe that their children's "problems" were not of the "ordinary" variety. In other words, parents evaluated the situation by comparing themselves and their children to other people. Here, too, expert claims played a role because parents compared their children to the non-specific, "normal" children they read about in child rearing manuals. Lauren adopted her twin daughters when they were just infants. They are now ten years old and thought to have developmental delays. Lauren recalled,

> I went and bought all kind of baby development books, and "Oh, they should be doing this at this age, and this at that age" . . . then, very quickly realizing that raising twins is slightly different than raising a singleton, I bought lots of twin books and read about twins. And [at first] they were making all their developmental milestones. . . . They started making sounds and appearing to communicate at three months. But at two [years old] they didn't talk a lot. They had maybe a vocabulary of five to ten words, which is not very much. So I questioned the pediatrician.

Parents also compared siblings to one another, and children's "symptoms" were brought into stark contrast when measured against the behaviors of a brother or sister. When describing his six-year-old son's aggression and disobedience, which emerged when the boy was four years old, Peter noted, "[Our other son's] temperament and behavior, his ability to cope with direction and discipline . . . it's just entirely different from [his brother]." Similarly, Paula, whose eight-year-old son was diagnosed with attention deficit/hyperactivity disorder when he was five, realized how challenging her son's behavior was when she had his younger sister. She recalled,

> The interesting thing is I never really realized how much I manage him, supervise him, or predict his next behavior until I had my daughter with me solo. And it's different with her. She's not ADHD . . . she's wonderful. . . . [When I'm

with my son], I always have to explain to him what the next step is for fear of his explosiveness or his rigidity or his obsessiveness . . . [and my daughter] just kind of goes along with the program, I don't have to tell her beforehand what's the next step.

Some parents used children's previous selves as points of comparison, and sudden changes in behavior often led them to seek help. Grace became worried about her daughter—who was eventually identified as having attention deficit/hyperactivity disorder—when her grades started to drop in junior high school. She explained, "[My daughter] did really good in elementary school . . . and then in seventh went to a public junior high. And she'd always gotten very good grades. And then all the sudden, probably about November in seventh-grade . . . she had D minuses, a couple of them." As noted earlier, Steve became increasingly suspicious about his daughter's behavior when she expressed a desire to quit her high school water polo team. He recalled, "Her water polo season kicked in. She was a good player on a very good team . . . she had hoped to play at the next level, and still does. She was a week or so into that, [and she started saying], 'I hate water polo. I hate that [coach], he's an asshole. I don't like those girls anymore.'" It was six months later that Steve and his wife discovered that their seventeen-year-old daughter was a cocaine addict.

Finally, parents used themselves as points of comparison, sometimes reflecting on their own childhood experiences. Susan's daughter was sixteen years old at the time of our interview. She suffers from trichotillomania ("the hair pulling disease"), is identified as gifted, has learning disabilities, and has had trouble in school since kindergarten. Susan said that she worried about her daughter when she thought about what she, herself, was like in high school. She said,

[My daughter is] not extremely popular. She doesn't have a ton of friends. I had tons and tons of friends. I straddled every group that there was at my high school. . . . I'm not trying to suggest that I'm anything special. . . . I wasn't homecoming queen, I wasn't anything like that. I just had lots of friends. And so did my [older daughter]. So when I look at [my younger daughter], I want that for her . . . she's very socially behind.

Mothers and fathers also compared themselves to other parents with similar aged children. Mike, whose eight-year-old son was diagnosed with ADHD when he was five, said that he became sharply aware of his son's "problematic" behaviors when he observed how easy it was for other parents to manage their children. He said, "Seeing our situation and getting together with other families, it [was] like, 'God, they're not having to work this damn hard!'"

THE CORROBORATION OF OTHERS

Though anxious parenting, mother-blame, biomedical discourse, and social comparisons directed parents' interpretive processes, key "turning points" tended to occur during interactions with friends, family members, and experts. Third party interpretation and intervention play a key role in determining whether or not trouble "exists" and, if it does, what kind of trouble it is.[17] Anna had noticed that her two-year-old daughter, now twenty-four and developmentally delayed, was not acquiring language. However, it was not until someone else suggested that she seek medical evaluation that she really began to think there might be an "underlying problem." She recalled, "When [my daughter] was two-and-a-half, a neighbor mentioned [that] maybe I should get her hearing tested. And I thought, 'Oooh, maybe other people are noticing it now too.' And I thought, 'It's not just me.' Because I began to notice it when she was two." In many cases, parents' suspicions were confirmed when their children's behaviors or conditions garnered the attention of schoolteachers or school officials. Mary and Phil's seventeen-year-old son was diagnosed with ADHD when he was in the sixth-grade and he began using and selling drugs three years prior to our interview. As an adolescent, Mary and Phil's son had been displaying deviant behavior for a few years, but it did not become clear that there were "real problems" until the school began sanctioning him in earnest. Phil said,

[Mary and I] were always, I think, a little concerned. [But] I put it off more to—as I told you earlier—[a] boy being a boy. Being one of these hyper kids who has no great love of school and does what he has to. It wasn't until really his freshman year . . . that we really started to get some inkling of, "There's some real deep issues here." . . . His first year of high school . . . he got in some trouble and missed the first day, [and] I think we were nervous from that point forward. And then the start of the sophomore year, . . . he [got into three] fights and was expelled right around Thanksgiving.

Not all of the parents I interviewed experienced such definitive turning points, but, like Mary and Phil, many discussed specific events that facilitated a sea change in their definitions of the situation. Some parents' suspicions culminated during semi-public gatherings that they used as narrative landmarks when telling their stories. For example, Keith and Valerie's daughter, who was eleven years old at the time of our interview, was diagnosed with autism when she was five; they decided to have their daughter evaluated after a holiday gathering where a family member remarked on her slow development of language. Keith recalled,

[Our daughter] was basically running around all day and never said anything. And [Valerie] and I had this feeling that something wasn't right. [One of our relatives]—shortly after that—said, "I think there's something going on with [your daughter]. She's not talking, guys. You need to do something about it." She was probably a little pushier than that because that was kind of her personality. . . . So that was right around when we kind of figured something was going on.

Similarly, Jessica and Peter, whose six-year-old son has undiagnosed behavioral problems that first manifested when he was four years old, sought help shortly after two parents of a fellow student attempted (unsuccessfully) to have their son expelled from his preschool. The boy had been hurting other children. Peter explained,

As we entered into a more structured environment there with [our son], probably the demands on him to interact with other children and adults there were a little more focused. . . . I think it became apparent to us that there was something that was more profound going on with him. . . . That's really when we first started seeking out some more, you know, focused, professional help. . . . It came to a point when there was actually a request that [he] leave the preschool. . . . That's maybe the most traumatic episode of it.

Whether it was a neighbor, teacher, or family member who corroborated parents' suspicions that something might be seriously wrong, these moments were significant because they were public. Once confirmed by other people, parents' private anxieties turned into "real" concerns. If they had not already sought expert advice, these moments of substantiation led them to do so.

LABELS, DIAGNOSES, AND PERSISTENT UNCERTAINTY

In the idealized medical encounter, the patient presents a particular set of "symptoms," and the doctor confidently supplies a clear diagnosis and appropriate treatment. Medical sociologists demonstrate that expert consultations quite often fall short of this expectation.[18] Nonetheless, once they decided to seek a professional evaluation, approximately half of the participants I interviewed had swift, unproblematic first encounters with medical or educational professionals. Sam and Grace's story unfolded in textbook-like fashion. They took Naomi (now seventeen) to see a psychologist in the sixth grade because she had not been turning in homework, had received several low grades, and a teacher suggested to Grace that they seek an evaluation. During the first visit, the psychologist diagnosed Naomi with attention deficit disorder. I asked Sam about his first impressions, and he replied,

Some of [our] first reactions were "Aha! That explains many things," and "Yes, that certainly sounds like a lot of what we're seeing, what we're experiencing. How she behaves, how she looks at things." So it explained a lot. It opened up the doors to the lack of knowledge or understanding about why or what was happening. So it helped us understand a lot about that.

Steve and Marie, who discovered seventeen-year-old Margo's cocaine addiction six months prior to our interview, recounted a similarly straightforward, "aha" moment. They had been noticing changes in their daughter's behavior for months, but once they sought third-party intervention, it was quickly determined that she was addicted to cocaine. Margo had run out of money to purchase drugs and was experiencing withdrawal symptoms when she and Marie got into an argument. The conflict escalated, and, when Margo threatened to harm herself, Marie called 911. Marie recalled what happened at the hospital,

I'm sitting in this room, [and] they come and they interview me. "Is she using any drugs?" I said, "Not to my knowledge, but I don't know! She could be!" . . . I said, "To be honest with you, that would answer a lot, but I have no idea." . . . And so they brought her in, and [the doctor] said, "Okay . . . you want to tell your mother something. . . . Here's your opportunity." And [my daughter] looked at me, she started crying, and she said, "I'm addicted to cocaine."

The moment of diagnosis was often the key turning point. For some, everything changed the moment an expert named their child's "problem." For example, Tim and Eve were already aware that their son—then a toddler but eighteen at the time of our interview—had some type of developmental delay when they requested that doctors test him for Fragile X syndrome. The positive test results were devastating, stripping them of the hope that their son would "catch up" to other children.

When we sat in the room with the people from their genetics department and they told us the results of the test and everything, even though we knew before that meeting, but they gave us the formal rundown. They were very matter of fact. I can't say that they were cold, per se, but in my opinion it was very like, "And your car needs a tune up and an oil change and your kid has Fragile X syndrome." And they were basically, "Don't expect him to be any smarter, ever, than an eight- or ten-year-old." And it was just really this kind of pronouncement of gloom and doom. And it was devastating. It was truly devastating.

Although receiving a clear label or diagnosis was sometimes shocking, and almost always painful, parents also experienced relief. Official labels are often double-edged in this way. They can be heartbreaking but also comforting insofar as they provide people with a clear interpretive framework to make sense of behaviors and conditions that had been formerly inexplicable.[19] They also indicate particular courses of treatment. When I asked Steve about his initial reaction to news of his daughter's addiction, he replied, "I would say number one, 'Well that sure explains a lot' . . . and number two, 'What do we do about it? *What* do we do about it?'" Nine days later, Steve and Marie put Margo on a plane to Utah, where she would spend six months in a therapeutic boarding program designed for teens with substance abuse "problems."

As Steve and Marie's situation illustrates, parents wanted professional validation, even in cases of traditionally non-medicalized or partially medicalized conditions, because it legitimated certain courses of action. At the time of our interview, Diane's daughter was twenty-one years old, un-partnered, and pregnant. When she was just fourteen, she began drinking, staying out at all hours, dating adult men, and getting poor grades. Even though Diane did not strongly frame her daughter's "problems" in terms of medical or psychological impairment, she sought the advice of doctors and therapists before making the decision to send her daughter to a wilderness camp.

> Before I ever sent her to the wilderness, I had checked with her original therapist, the therapist I had been working with, her pediatrician. . . . I had her entirely psychologically reviewed with a battery of tests and everything. And everybody agreed, "This girl . . . if you don't send her, she's really lost."

At the same time, not all parents were receptive to professionals' assessments of their children's "problems." For example, Paula, whose son was eight years old at the time of our interview, was very resistant to a psychologist's opinion that her son, then five years old, had attention deficit disorder. She had sought the help of an expert who had written books about "strong-willed" children, and she expected that the doctor would label her son in these terms. Regarding the ADD diagnosis, she recalled thinking, "Here's another child being mislabeled and misdiagnosed." In the year following the diagnosis, however, her son's behavior worsened. After experimenting with different discipline strategies and reluctantly agreeing to try medication, her views on attention deficit disorder shifted. She explained,

> [Now] I see genetically where it comes from . . . when he responded with [the medication]. When we exhausted all the behavioral stuff, and I thought, "Okay, well there's obviously something more to this than just behavioral issues and parenting issues." Because no matter what I did or what I didn't do, there was no difference in his behavior. So I believe there is an organic cause.

Unlike Paula, a few parents received diagnoses that did not "stick." As discussed in the previous chapter, Sergio and Joan's fifteen-year-old son, Nathan, began showing symptoms of mental illness when he was eleven, and doctors think he may develop schizophrenia. Nathan was diagnosed with ADHD more than once, but Sergio and Joan were convinced that this was a mistake. Sergio explained,

> We just kept going to doctors, doctors. And he's had so many different diagnoses, like ADHD, or whatever, and he doesn't have that. . . . We got to the point where we were going to doctors in San Francisco on a weekly basis, just to find the best [care] for our son. And we found someone that again was going back to ADHD, whatever, and we knew it wasn't that.

Parents in this situation often continued to search for doctors until they found someone whose opinions were more closely aligned with their own.

The "ideal" medical encounter notwithstanding, uncertainty is as much a part of the medical enterprise as it is a feature of people's lived experiences of illness.[20] When doctors do not know what is happening, clinical uncertainty exacerbates patients' own existential uncertainties.[21] Thus, parents had a particularly difficult time when experts agreed that something was wrong but were unable to name "the problem." Such was the case for Bill, whose son (now sixteen) began having seizures when he was five-months-old. He recalled his frustration:

> The doctors never used the word "epilepsy" with us. They always said, "A seizure disorder, a seizure disorder." They never ever said, "Your son is epileptic." . . . And it's like, "Just say it! Tell me something so I can hang on, just don't give me some general fluff term!" We wanted a diagnosis. We wanted a reason. All parents want a reason so you can at least start from there and do some researching and kind of go and learn and stuff. Otherwise, you know, just undiagnosed seizure disorder.

Prolonged periods of uncertainty following expert consultation were common across problem type. Lauren's adopted, twin, ten-year-old daughters have learning problems and poorly defined disabilities. Lauren, who first became concerned about their development when they were three, recounted her experiences.

> We went from an original diagnosis of being at risk for mental retardation to just, we don't know. They now say [my first daughter] has ADHD. They aren't even sure what [my second daughter's] problems are, other than they both have a severe language disorder . . . one of the doctors told me we're in the forty percent category of "science hasn't caught up with it yet."

Parents without specific labels or diagnoses were unsure about which treatments might help their children, and they lacked the clarity that specific names could provide. Frustration was a recurring theme among the parents in this group. Peter's six-year-old son has trouble controlling his emotions and is aggressive with other children. These problems first manifested when he was four years old. Peter's son had not yet received a diagnosis, and he commented,

> It's frustrating having something where it's difficult to diagnose . . . not knowing how to treat it. What are the right interventions? Are there different medications or therapies or services, or something that we should be having for him? I think that's probably the biggest thing. And I guess also at the same time, there's the issue of just psychologically wanting to understand what we were coping with.

Including Bill, Lauren, and Peter, twelve of the families in this study had not yet received a specific label or diagnosis for their children's "problems." Although these parents longed for more specific explanations, the mere confirmation from professionals that something was wrong provided some reassurance. This was particularly true among mothers who had had a difficult time convincing others of their children's "problems." Peter's spouse, Jessica, said that expert validation had been essential to gaining support. Her sister, who thought "the problem" was lenient parenting, adopted Jessica's biomedical definition of the situation once doctors suspected mental illness. Jessica said, "[Now] it's not just me telling [my sister] that there's some neurological, biological thing going on. It's like, this is finally somebody [else], an expert."

Some parents lacked any sort of professional validation, at least at first, and their situations may have been the most challenging of all. In a handful of cases, experts initially told parents that their children did not have "significant problems." Carol, whose thirteen-year-old son was diagnosed with Asperger's syndrome when he was four, gradually became angry at doctors' unwillingness to consider the possibility that something might be wrong. She said,

> [I was] upset with the doctors patting me on the shoulder and telling me it's gonna be okay. And I was always an early intervention person. In fact, for nine years I was a parent-infant specialist, trying to give kids early intervention to give them a good start. And so I was actually spittin' mad at the doctors that kept blowing me off.

Similarly, Rhonda and Seth sought help from their fourteen-year-old daughter's therapist when she ran away from home and was living on the streets. Their daughter is now nineteen, living at home, and no longer using drugs. During our interview, they had the following exchange.

RHONDA: We were getting, at the time, no support at all from the therapist . . . because we were saying, "We need advice . . . ."

SETH: "What can we do here?" . . . And [the therapist is] worse than useless! She's not helping us at all. In fact, she's telling us everything is okay! It's like, "What are you talking about?"

It is not that parents wished their children to be diagnosed or labeled as having significant "problems." However, once their interactions with family members, friends, or teachers had encouraged them to define children's "symptoms" as "problematic" enough to require expert intervention, they wanted an explanation and a remedy. Although the confirmation of medical professionals provided some parents with a sense of relief, most of the parents in this study—even those whose children received clear diagnoses—later found that understanding children's "problems," much less "fixing" them, was not as straightforward as a simple visit to the doctor or psychologist. In many cases, uncertainty became a somewhat permanent feature of daily living.

Quantitative data suggests that the numbers of "problem children" in the United States are growing. Autism is on the rise,[22] doctors and psychologists diagnose more children with mental health "problems" and learning "disabilities" than ever before,[23] and a highly lucrative industry dedicated to the rehabilitation of middle-class teenaged addicts continues to grow.[24] This chapter provides a glimpse into some of the micro-social processes that contribute to these larger trends. I contend here that deep anxiety about childrearing, an intensive orientation to mothering and pervasive mother-blame, and biomedical accounts of human development prime parents to interpret children's conditions and behaviors as "problematic." Because these contexts shape late-modern parenthood in the broadest sense, even those who do not come to see their children as "problem children" might find their own experiences reflected in parents' early suspicions. However, the emergence of trouble is contingent upon a number of factors, including parents' own familiarity and comfort with biomedical discourse, a series of social comparisons, and some degree of third-party corroboration. Though these factors were neither determinative nor sequential, their presence created a perfect storm out of which turning points were likely to emerge. Indeed, parents' understandings of their children and themselves shifted as they came to view their situations as "seriously troublesome."

It is tempting to view parents' troubles as having started with a particular "problem"—a child's learning disability, addiction, or seizure disorder, for example—that went on to upset various aspects of daily life. In truth, the relationship between "problems" and disruption is not so cut-and-dried. In most cases, parents were coming to view their children as having "significant problems" *at the same time* that other aspects of their lives were coming undone. By the time most parents sought professional evaluations, children's "problematic" conditions and behaviors had already started to play havoc with routine interactions. As some of the previous quotes indicate, early conflicts about how to define situations unsettled parents' relationships with one another, family members, and friends. In fact, disrupted routines, relationships, expectations, and selves—the topics of subsequent chapters—helped to both generate and reinforce the view that children's conditions and behaviors were seriously "problematic."

Nonetheless, the social "realization" of trouble was significant because, in most cases, it led to further trouble. The acknowledgment that something was wrong meant that something needed to be done. As I discuss in the next chapter, this launched most of the mothers in this study into an all-encompassing and exhausting search for effective remedies. Somewhat paradoxically, the quest for treatments disrupted the time-order of the families' daily activities to such an extent that, in some cases, it was far more troubling than children's initial conditions or behaviors. Furthermore, existential uncertainty haunted parents long after they had landed upon satisfactory labels or reasonable courses of treatment. These parents had identified their children as being "out of character" or "out of place."[25] As meaningful anchors for parents' own selves, the disruption of children's identities left their mothers and fathers feeling as though there was little they could be sure of.

3 • ELUSIVE REMEDIES AND DISRUPTED ROUTINES

Claire is a doctoral student working on her dissertation. She is also the mother of two boys, a job that takes priority over her academic pursuits. "I'm just really into [my kids]," she explained, as we sipped tea at her dining room table. "That's way more important than my PhD . . . my main identity is as a mother, without a doubt." Her younger son, Andrew, was two years old when his temperament changed. He had been an "easy baby" aside from some sleeping problems, but suddenly he "stopped gaining words [and] started crying a lot more. He became much more introverted. His eyes looked clouded, and his language just didn't go anywhere." Claire eventually sought their pediatrician's advice, and Andrew had just turned three when doctors diagnosed him with autism. Claire then leapt into action.

> I immediately got in contact with CAI, the Coalition for Autism Intervention[1] . . . . They're a very powerful group . . . one of the most powerful in the country. . . . That's when things really started to move. . . . They're extremely aggressive [and] they're very wealthy. . . . They've got a lot of research behind them . . . so I found out about home programs. . . . I found out how *outrageously* expensive they are. I found out how you get funding. I found out about the special diet many kids are on. I found out about a million things.

Claire postponed her graduate work and, with the help of CAI, fought to get funding from the state to implement an intensive home program for her son. She turned one of her bedrooms into a therapy room and spent the next two years working with behavioral, speech, and occupational therapists trying to improve her son's condition. When Andrew entered kindergarten at their local public school, Claire resumed her studies but remained intensively involved in his education. She ensured that Andrew's classroom aide was trained by the organization that had administered his home program. Later, when she believed he was not receiving the help he needed, she persuaded school officials to pay for outside professionals who provided further assistance in the classroom. When I interviewed Claire, she had recently enrolled Andrew in a private school for children with special needs and had hired a lawyer to compel the school district to cover the tuition. She was candid about these efforts. She said, "There's a certain amount of dollars out there, right? So what do you do as a parent? You decide, I'm really sorry that not all the kids are gonna get these good services, but mine is."

Though Claire believed that advocacy and intensive therapy were absolutely necessary for treating her son's autism, her work on his behalf came at a price. At the end of the interview, when I asked Claire if she had any advice for other parents of children with autism, she replied,

> You have to take care of your child, and you have to take care of yourself . . . [With autism] you have to move quickly, and you have to get a home program in place . . . get it established before the age of three. So you almost have to postpone taking care of yourself in that situation. Because you do need to get some counseling or a support group or something like that as well. Which I didn't do. Because I was fighting, you know? I just fought, fought, fought . . . I didn't [take care of myself] at all.

This chapter is about how parents' efforts to identify, manage, and remedy children's problems displaced other activities and upended day-to-day routines. Like Claire, most of the mothers—and many of the fathers—in this study reapportioned their time and energy so that they could focus on helping their children. In many cases, this required them to marginalize or "postpone" activities that contributed to their own well-being. Exercise, healthful eating, and sleep were jettisoned to the periphery of parents' attentions as children's problems became the primary focus of daily life. In most cases, the day-to-day, hands-on management of children's conditions and behaviors was enough to upset parents' routines. However, as Claire's story highlights, parents' efforts to secure medical and educational resources for their children compounded disruption. Somewhat paradoxically, finding and financing the treatments that women deemed necessary tended to create more disruption than the conditions and behaviors they sought to remedy.

The stories that drive this chapter strongly feature what Arthur Frank calls the "restitution narrative."[2] Their plotlines hinge on the assumption that proper identification and treatment will ameliorate, if not fix, children's problems. This feature of parents' stories must be understood in light of how children's problems impacted parents themselves; women's efforts were all at once meant to help their children *and* to manage the conflict and uncertainty described in the previous chapter. Women had a tremendous stake in remedying children's problems, but medical uncertainty and the proliferation of information about children's health meant that most "problems" had countless potential names and just as many remedies. Looking for answers, women waded into a sea of scientific and pseudo-scientific claims and set out to navigate the rough waters of medical and educational bureaucracies. Whatever success these efforts might have had in helping children, they provided women with a sense of purpose and momentum at a time when the meaning of what was happening to them, their children, and their families was otherwise elusive.

The work that mothers did to garner institutional support adheres to the ideology of intensive motherhood, to be sure. For some, children's advocacy was an all-encompassing endeavor, organized by children's needs and underpinned by the belief that mothers are the only ones who can make sure those needs are met. However, the concept of "concerted cultivation" more aptly captures their efforts. As middle-class economic prospects have dwindled, parents have become increasingly shrewd about maximizing children's opportunities for success. Instead of believing that children will develop "naturally" if they are safe and loved, parents assume that they must actively *cultivate* children's intellectual, physical, and emotional well-being.[3] Mediating children's experiences in institutional settings is an important feature of concerted cultivation, and middle-class mothers play a key role in shaping what happens in the classroom.[4]

If parenting "ordinary" children requires concerted cultivation, parenting children with "problems" requires nothing less than vigilantism.[5] Mothers whose children have problems can be said to enact "a cutting-edge model of concerted cultivation."[6] In this neoliberal era of limited public assistance and a strong rhetoric of personal responsibility, they go above and beyond the already taxing demands of contemporary childrearing. As I will demonstrate in this chapter, they do so at a steep personal cost. My data also suggest that the type of problem a child has strongly shapes women's experiences in institutional settings. Relative to other groups of parents, the mothers of school-aged children with invisible or ostensibly controversial disabilities had to fight much harder to garner medical and educational resources. They became particularly consumed by the demands of advocating for their children.

DAY-TO-DAY CARE

As I discussed in the introduction, caring for children in our late-modern, Western society is a time- and energy-intensive task, even in the best of circumstances. Children's problems further intensified the routine demands of parenthood. When children required ongoing medical attention, their mothers and fathers became their doctors and nurses. Parents whose children had learning disabilities became teachers, and those whose children had emotional problems became therapists. For example, Bill's sixteen-year-old son developed a seizure disorder when he was five months old, and he now has developmental disabilities. Years ago, a neurologist had charged Bill with charting the details of his son's seizures. During bad periods the little boy had several each day. Here Bill describes the task.

> We really had to plan and keep a journal on a calendar so we [could] plot the seizure activity. I did a lot of the note-takings during the seizures and stuff . . . just trying to keep track of everything. Which way did his head turn? . . . did his head turn right, did his head turn left? Did his eyes go right, left? Was it the left side of his body shaking, just his arms or a leg? . . . did it kind of march up and down his body? During the two-minute seizure, did it start with his arms and move to the full body? Was it just a blank-stare seizure?

While parents like Bill learned how to follow medical protocol, parents like Martha, whose thirteen-year-old daughter has learning disabilities and has struggled in school since kindergarten, tried to implement programs that would help their children perform better in school.

> [The teacher would] give me the ideas, and I'd come home and do them. You know, the sticker thing, the discipline thing, a certain homework hour . . . and, "Make sure you get her in sports. She needs a sport . . . don't make it a lonely sport . . . make it an involved sport so she gets in with other kids . . ." [And,] "Get her in Girl Scouts," you know, "Girl Scouts, where girls grow strong" . . . [and I would say] "Okay, okay, we're goin', we're doin' it!"

When children had drug and alcohol problems and were delinquent or truant, parents spent extra time trying to monitor them and keep track of their whereabouts. Andrea's daughter has had drug and alcohol problems since the tenth-grade. She was diagnosed with depression in junior high school and has also been in trouble for fighting. Andrea recalled how difficult it had been when her daughter, now nineteen, still lived at home.

> I'd be calling the police at two A.M. in the morning saying, "I don't know where my daughter is" I was a crazy woman . . . writing down phone numbers, trying to pick up [and] listen in on her conversations to find out who she's hanging out with. . . . I was scouring the libraries for reading material, and all kinds of things. I [was] going to school everyday, checking on attendance, etcetera, etcetera. I mean, the attendance people I think felt sorry for me because I was there every day.

Across the spectrum of problem types, managing children's conditions and behaviors consumed parents. For those whose children had traditional disabilities, the intensive work of caring for a young child was prolonged indefinitely. For Sarah and Matt, it was like caring for an infant, year after year. Sarah's thirteen-year-old biological son was diagnosed with cerebral palsy at birth and is severely disabled.

SARAH: I need to get away from the home to get rest . . . [my son with disabilities] still wakes up at five or so. And so I'm just not getting enough sleep . . .

MATT: And also kind of being aware of someone's every move . . . as a young parent, you're very in tune with a baby . . . you're in tune to those changes. And eventually the kid is out of diapers . . . [and] to a certain degree your level of fear and involvement and all those kinds of things kind of goes down.

SARAH: The kid becomes more independent.

MATT: They can wake up, they can put their clothes on by themselves . . . so the parents can kind of sleep in . . .

SARAH: But with [our younger son] . . . you can't do that.

The work of managing the emotions of children with mental health problems was no less draining. At different times in the past ten years, Amanda's son has been diagnosed with attention deficit/hyperactivity disorder, dyslexia, and bipolar disorder. Amanda regularly spends hours with her fifteen-year-old son, talking through his violent outbursts and episodes of depression.

[When my son is upset] I have to keep reminding him about how much I love him, and keep reminding him about what a great kid he is. And I have found that positive reinforcement has been the best thing for him. He will start to immediately get down on himself, and he immediately will start criticizing himself and going into a very negative mode once he's done something that he's remorseful about. And it's a matter of then trying to head that off and stop it. And bring him back up to a place where he feels good about himself again. And sometimes it takes, you know, an hour, sometimes it takes three or four hours.

In all but a few cases, women spent more time than fathers doing the day-to-day work associated with children's problems. However, children's conditions and behaviors often led fathers to become more hands-on with their parenting. For example, Mike, whose eight-year-old son was diagnosed with attention deficit/hyperactivity disorder when he was five, said that he had to become more of a disciplinarian because of his son's behavioral problems; he did this deliberately because it did not feel "natural."

[Our son's problems have] really forced me to step up . . . in terms of being a dad, being the authority figure and not just sitting back and letting my wife [take care of everything]. . . . I have to consciously do that at times. . . . I have to go, "Okay, don't just sit back and wait for [Paula] to respond, get up and take care of it."

Many fathers had to become more involved because mothers simply could not manage everything on their own. Jessica and Peter's six-year-old son has trouble controlling his emotions and is aggressive with other children. These problems first manifested when he was four years old. Peter gave Jessica respite on nights and weekends.

We felt pushed to our limits often. . . . My work was the kind that it's hard for me to get away from it. So what that meant is more that I maybe give her breaks [on] nights or weekends and give her some time off. Some time to go do things . . . definitely at those kind of breaking points . . . it would just kind of build up to an extreme level. . . . At least when we were both there, one of us could say, "I just need a break from this," and the other one would step in.

As I discuss in more detail in the next section, the dramatic expansion of parenting at home served to diminish other aspects of parents' daily lives. Nonetheless, women's efforts to advocate for children in medical and educational settings often overshadowed the demands of hands-on care.

ADVOCACY CARE

There is a conceptual distinction between "direct carework," or the "interventions, routines, and patterns related to the actual care of the child," and what scholars call "advocacy carework."[7] The latter term refers to how, in addition to the hands-on management of children's conditions and behaviors, mothers work hard to secure medical and educational resources on children's behalf. Most of the mothers I interviewed performed some type of advocacy carework, and their efforts to procure particular diagnoses, treatments, and school accommodations placed additional strain on family routines that were, in many cases, already precarious.

Doctors' visits played havoc with parents' schedules, particularly when mothers, fathers, or medical professionals disagreed about the nature of children's "problems." As I mentioned in the previous chapter, parents who lacked professional validation or received unsatisfactory diagnoses sought second, third, and fourth opinions in an effort to achieve clarity. In these cases, mothers spent time on the phone getting referrals, scheduling appointments, and driving—sometimes long distances—to have their children evaluated by specialists. The sheer busyness of so many consultations was reflected in parents' interviews. Convinced that Nathan had a serious mental health "problem," Joan repeatedly rejected doctors' assertions that he had attention deficit disorder. Sergio, who did not initially believe that their son had a "problem" at all, commented, "We just kept going to doctors. . . . I mean, we got to the point where we were going to doctors on a weekly basis." Similarly, Jen and Carl spent years trying to figure out what was "wrong" with their second adopted daughter. The girl was eight years old at the time of our interview and is now thought to have fetal alcohol effects. Like Joan and Sergio, they saw doctor after doctor:

CARL: We went to how many doctors? I can't even explain to you how many doctors . . .

JEN: Nine.

CARL: How many therapists . . .

JEN: I kept every card.

CARL: Just to where, I don't even know who's doing what anymore! And no one is telling us anything!

Uncertainty fueled busyness, and there was a strong relationship between "not knowing" and women's advocacy carework. The less agreement there was about children's "problems" or how to treat them, the more time mothers spent on the Internet, in libraries, and on the phone searching for answers. Sergio's wife Joan, recalling the months she spent trying to find out what was wrong with her son, said, "I was researching, and I was calling, and I was going, going, going all the time . . . and I just would read every study I could find. I subscribed to different psychiatry bulletins so that I get the latest information."

Women whose children had drug and alcohol problems spent less time than other mothers doing advocacy carework. This may have been because addiction is only partly medicalized and, as I discuss in the next chapter, people were more apt to hold teenaged children culpable for their own problems. However, mothers in this situation did sometimes immerse themselves in information about potential treatment options. Seth and Rhonda's daughter, now nineteen, sober, and living at home, began abusing drugs and ran away when she was fourteen. When Rhonda and Seth realized that their daughter's therapist could not help them, they took matters into their own hands. They decided they would take their daughter, against her will, to an out-of-state treatment facility. Here, Rhonda describes her research.

On my end, I'm calling different people and talking with different people. I'm calling different institutions trying to get a feeling. I'm looking on the Internet. I'm looking at different things that are telling me something about the character of these programs, something about who's behind the programs, telling me something about what the philosophy is behind it. You know, all those kinds of things. And then I did talk with some educational [consultants].

As noted in the previous chapter, women had a greater stake than men in the identification and treatment of children's "problems." For them, the anxiety of not knowing was amplified by the ever-present threat of mother-blame. Advocacy carework helped mothers to seize power and bring meaning to uncertain situations that threatened their identities as "good" mothers. For example, research allowed some women to secure medical labels. When I asked Jen and Carl how Becca came to be diagnosed with an attachment disorder as a toddler, Jen replied, "Actually, I found it on the Internet, is what happened. I, like, typed in the symptoms. 'Cause it was so frustrating not to know what was going on! And it was clear that that's what it was." After consulting with an attachment specialist, Becca received a formal attachment disorder diagnosis. Like Jen, several women did extensive research, diagnosed their own children, and then set out to find like-minded doctors. When recalling how her twenty-five-year-old son came to be diagnosed with attention deficit disorder in the sixth-grade, Judy said,

> I went to [a meeting for parents of children with attention deficit disorder] to . . . see if [Jason] really might [have ADD], or maybe not, or whatever. . . . The group was very active and very big at that time. They used to have seminars. They're wonderful! [They] have speakers come in. . . . So that's when I thought, "This is what's going on here with this child!"

Healthcare in the United States positions doctors as go-betweens who manage the interests of insurance and pharmaceutical companies on the one hand and the interests of healthcare consumers on the other. This limits doctors' power and makes patients themselves key players in the processes of medicalization.[8] The diminished power of medical professionals and the redefinition of patients as "consumers" encourages the kind of advocacy carework described here. The availability of the Internet, especially, allows for savvy and informed patients to self-diagnose and "shop" for amenable physicians.[9] The contemporary politics of special education further help to explain the demands of advocacy care, particularly among the mothers of school-aged children with invisible or ill-defined disabilities.

THE SPECIAL CASE OF INVISIBLE AND ILL-DEFINED DISABILITIES

In 1975, the federal government passed legislation ensuring a free and appropriate education for all children with disabilities. The Individuals with Disabilities Education Act (IDEA) requires public schools to meet the needs of all eligible children, free of charge, and in the least restrictive environment possible. Provisions vary widely, ranging from curb cuts for students in wheelchairs, to interpreters for children who are deaf, to personal tutors for children with learning disabilities. Accommodations for children with special needs can include laptop computers, extra time on exams, personal note-takers, and alternative disciplinary measures when children misbehave.[10] Because special education is a legal mandate, parents can sue schools for not providing their children with necessary services. As Claire's case demonstrates, parents can demand that the state pay for private education when the local public schools are not meeting their children's needs.

The proportion of children eligible for special education in the United States has increased markedly since the implementation of IDEA, growing from 3.7 million in 1976–1977 to 6.1 million in 1999–2000.[11] In large part, this is because the criteria used to determine which students are eligible for special education has broadened significantly since 1975. Children between the ages of three and five are now eligible for services and accommodations, as are students diagnosed with attention deficit disorder and autism.[12] Furthermore, 38 percent of the children receiving special education in the United States are categorized as having learning disabilities in specific subject areas, such as reading or mathematics,[13] and there are no universally accepted standards for determining the presence or absence of such disabilities.[14] It is possible that the growth of special education is due, in part, to diagnostic expansion.

Although special education accounts for approximately 20 percent of U.S. spending on primary and secondary education,[15] some scholars have characterized our era as one of "public stinginess."[16] On average, the per-student cost of special education is approximately twice that of regular education,[17] and because the federal government covers only a fraction of the money necessary to provide special services, states and local school districts shoulder most of those costs.[18] This means that parents seeking special education compete for resources at the local level, and school officials must apportion limited funds. Indeed, most of the parents in this study who sought special education characterized school officials as tight-fisted.

The political context described here selectively encouraged some mothers to engage in advocacy carework more than others. More specifically, mothers whose school-aged children had invisible or ill-defined disorders were particularly likely to have adversarial relationships with medical professionals and school personnel who they believed stood between their children and necessary labels and accommodations.[19] This group of mothers enacted their cultural capital in a number of ways: they did extensive research in order to facilitate and counter expert claims, frequently prepared for and attended school meetings where they had to argue their cases, and sought the help of mediators, child advocates, and lawyers when negotiating with school personnel. Carol, whose thirteen-year-old son was diagnosed with Asperger's syndrome when he was four, was one such mother. As noted in the previous chapter, Carol had been concerned about her son's behavior since he was toddler. He seemed highly sensitive and anti-social, and she had visited numerous doctors in an attempt to determine the nature of his "problems." She was a teacher at the time and used her budding knowledge of autism to navigate the diagnostic process. She said,

> We were struggling with the doctors, and . . . it was really hard for me because . . . these people were the experts, and I was just the mother and the teacher. . . . To make a long story short, I got my first [child with] Asperger's in class . . . [and] it began to slowly hit me. . . . I was going, "Oh my god. This is my child." And so it was very hard because I couldn't get him diagnosed and I kept trying to find people [who agreed with me]. . . . I did go back to some of the doctors who had diagnosed some other thing, and some of the other therapists. I mean, we had a whole list of them. . . . I went back to them and showed them the diagnosis. I said, "I just want you to know this."

Carol explained that receiving a diagnosis was important because it allowed her to focus on treatment. However, even with the Asperger's label, she had a difficult time getting the school to provide her son with the services she thought were necessary. She said, "I really struggled with the school district, trying to get services. And we've even talked to lawyers, and we've been very aggressive."

Even once educational accommodations were established, mothers whose children had invisible or ill-defined problems took an ongoing management role. For example, Grace, whose seventeen-year-old adopted daughter was diagnosed with attention deficit disorder in the sixth-grade and now also suffers from depression, met with school officials at least once a year to establish which services and accommodations her daughter would receive. She explained,

> Every year [her individual education plan] gets evaluated, and there's just certain things we put in there . . . and every year I learn a little bit more [about] what to put in there and what she needs. . . . Like, one year . . . I think our doctor said, "Put down that you need more time to take tests or you need additional time to turn something in."

Grace said that even when administrators consented to her requests, school-teachers were sometimes reluctant to provide the agreed-upon accommodations. Like Carol, who returned to previous doctors to inform them of her son's diagnosis, Grace tried to educate teachers about the nature of her daughter's problems.[20] She stated, "I bring in education to teach teachers sometimes because unless you have someone with [ADD] or know somebody with it [you don't understand]. I tell them, 'It's a neurological disorder . . . it's not a mental illness, it's not a disease, but it is something that's real.'"

Statements like these reveal the class-specific nature of women's advocacy care. It is not as though poor or working-class mothers do not fight for their children in institutional contexts; indeed they do.[21] However, research skills, extensive knowledge, and the air of authority displayed by women like Carol and Grace are clear examples of cultural capital, or the non-material resources afforded by their middle-class backgrounds. In fact, for some of the mothers in this study, advocacy care required so much specialized knowledge that they came to think of mothering as a "professional" endeavor. Worried that medical and educational professionals would blame them for children's problems or dismiss them as "overemotional" or "overbearing," some women crafted professional presentations of self to contend with the bureaucratic gatekeepers who controlled access to special services. Claire, whose nine-year-old son was diagnosed with autism when he was three, explained,

> You get emotional, right? Because you get really upset. I haven't lost it, but I know some mothers who really have. . . . [School personnel], they look at the mother [and think], "She's slightly mentally ill, and he's got autism, I wonder if there's a connection." (Laughs) I know that they think that! Because we're, like, on edge . . . I try to *not* appear that way in public with them, I try to appear together and professional.

Although mothers like Claire said that it was necessary to become assertive in order to secure medical and educational resources, some feared that if medical and educational professionals viewed them as too aggressive or overbearing, it could work against them.[22] Because over-involvement can mark women as "bad" mothers,[23] women worked to distance themselves from "pushy" parents. Jen, who regularly met with school personnel to discuss her second daughter's progress, described the predicament as follows: "It's really hard to work with the school community because if you're too much of a squeaky wheel, they don't like you, and that trickles down to your child. If you're not enough, they won't give you anything!"

As demonstrated here, when problems were invisible or ill-defined, women who sought accommodations had to convince medical and educational personnel that their children had legitimate special needs. Although most of the mothers in this study researched their children's "problems" and advocated for particular kinds of diagnoses and treatments, advocacy carework tended to consume the lives of mothers whose school-aged children had learning disabilities, autism spectrum disorders, or mental health problems.

THE BREAKDOWN OF ROUTINE AND CONSEQUENCES FOR PARENTS' WELL-BEING

As parents recounted the histories of their troubles, they described how children's problems came to occupy the center of family life. This was the case for all types of problem; due in part to advocacy carework, even conditions such as attention deficit/hyperactivity disorder became the primary focus of parents' attentions. Grace's spouse, Sam, explained, "[Naomi's attention deficit disorder is] probably the biggest, most consistent concern or issue in the whole household for all of us. . . . I mean, anything else is a distant second in terms of its influence or impact. There's been nothing else that has even come close to that for the two of us or the three of us, for me individually." Naomi was seventeen at the time of our interview and also suffers from depression.

The expansion of carework changed the temporal organization of parents' daily activities; with so much time and energy dedicated to managing children's problems, other obligations and interests fell by the wayside. Meals uncooked and houses unclean, the routines of domestic life were thrown off balance. Martha described how her evenings changed as her thirteen-year-old daughter's learning problems (which had started in kindergarten) became worse. She said, "I would read to her . . . 'cause she couldn't read! . . . she'd get home from school, we'd curl up on the couch and the bed. I mean, from a family point of view, there were lots of dinners that weren't made . . . [because] we had been reading for hours." The disruption of household order compounded parents' troubles, as Jessica explained. "The house gets kind of messy because I don't have much time to do it," she said, "and then it makes me more depressed, and everybody more depressed."

To make room for additional carework, many women adjusted their employment schedules. For example, Carol, whose thirteen-year-old son was diagnosed with Asperger's syndrome when he was four, quit her job so that she could spend more time and energy trying to helping her son. Here she recalls how the demands of carework became incompatible with the demands of being a schoolteacher.

The day that I really made my final decision [to quit my job], I was teaching a special [education] class, and I had some very medically fragile children. . . . I was gastro-tube feeding one of my students [when] . . . the phone rang in my room and [my son's] teacher called and said, "You have to come and get him right now." He was having a severe anxiety attack and he was just out of control . . . It was horrible. I mean, I thought, "I can't get to my son," I mean, they're calling and telling me to come and get him because he is so upset they can't control him, and I can't leave my medically fragile students.

While women whose children required moment-to-moment supervision and high levels of advocacy carework sometimes stopped working outside of the home altogether, mothers like Andrea reduced their hours. She said, "I did stop working full-time and only worked part-time. I made that change because I felt when [my daughter] was in junior high and went through the depressed period that I just need to be around more. . . . I only worked three days a week."

Intensive mothering practices leave women with a dearth of time for themselves.[24] Among the mothers I interviewed, the loss of "me-time" was so great that it had negative physical and psychological consequences. Whether they were attempting to monitor their teenagers' whereabouts or their toddlers' interactions with other children, parents—and especially mothers—said that attending to children's problems meant that they attended less often to their own needs. Mary, whose seventeen-year-old son began using and selling drugs three years ago, recalled how sleep became elusive as her son deepened his involvement with drugs and drug dealing. "I could hardly function," she said. "[Phil and I] never slept a whole night. I couldn't go to sleep. [Our son] was sneaking out, so every creak I heard, I would be sure that he was either coming in or going out. . . . Then he would run away . . . there was never any rest or peace of mind or peace at all."

Several women said that they could no longer make time for exercise. Paula's eight-year-old son was diagnosed with attention deficit/hyperactivity disorder when he was five, and when I asked her if motherhood was different than she imagined it would be, she laughed and replied,

[I thought] I'd be a lot thinner. It wasn't until recently that I went back to the gym, and that's because when I had [my son] at home with me, I could never take him to a place and leave him in the child care room, because he would be too aggressive.

Bill, who had become a stay-at-home father after his five-month-old son started having seizures, echoed these comments: "It's overwhelming. . . . You're not taking care of yourself. You're not eating right, you're not exercising, you're not sleeping. . . . My health deteriorated, was going downhill very fast."

As sleep, exercise, and healthy eating were pushed to the margins of parents' attentions, so went life's simple pleasures. Exhausted and overwhelmed by the demands of carework, parents felt as though children's problems cast a shadow over their entire lives. Peter, whose six-year-old son developed social and behavioral problems two years prior to our interview, commented, "There were plenty of days and nights when we were just kind of at the end of our rope dealing with this situation. And it didn't leave a lotta extra energy for having fun, you know? For just having light times or humor or romance. . . . It just more kind of wore us out, you know?" Judy made a similar remark about her teenaged son's attention deficit disorder. "I felt like it was with me all the time," she said. "I felt like this kid and his situation was at the forefront of my life almost all the time. . . . It kind of takes the joy out of life in general." Some of the parents I interviewed described periods of upheaval that stretched on for years. Their fatigue was profound. Sandra, whose thirteen-year-old adopted son has had ill-defined behavioral and mental health problems since birth, explained, "We've been doing this now for twelve-and-a-half years. . . . It is so exhausting . . . it's a very difficult way to live."

As evinced by the tendency of carework to marginalize other activities and unsettle the temporal organization of daily life, parents' troubles gained momentum in domino-like fashion. The emerging interpretation that children's conditions and behaviors were "seriously problematic" gave way to concerted efforts, usually on the part of mothers, to name and remedy those "problems." Through the disruption of routine, intensive carework carried children's problems into other areas of parents' lives, thereby amplifying their feelings of distress. In other words, efforts to fix the problem paradoxically served to amplify parents' troubles. As I discuss in the next chapter, trouble continued to grow and spill outward as the unsettling of daily routines disrupted parents' relationships with one another and with friends and family members.

My analysis so far highlights the pivotal part that mothers played in constructing and seeking solutions for children's problems. However, women's active posture should not be taken to mean that fathers were absent from or untouched by children's problems. Though women tended to pilot the interpretive and logistic processes described thus far, the fathers I interviewed also experienced uncertainty and discontinuity. As I discuss in the next two chapters, men were not invulnerable to stigma, nor were they impassive about their children's situations. On the contrary, most men were deeply pained by their children's problems. Nonetheless, the burden of concerted cultivation—or of vigilantism, particularly in the case of children with invisible or controversial problems—was disproportionately borne by mothers, thereby gendering the tenor of parents' troubles.

While the unsettling of participants' routines was, on the one hand, a practical matter of not having enough time to care for themselves, parents' narratives of exhaustion and joylessness suggest that there was an existential dimension to their woes. Patterns of time bring order to social life, and our sense of "okay-ness" relies on certain activities taking place at certain times and for certain amounts of time.[25] Medical anthropologist Gay Becker explains, "A sense of continuity is captured in ordinary routines of daily life, the mundane and the comforting sameness of repetitive activities, such as drinking a cup of coffee with the morning newspaper. These activities give structure and logic to people's lives."[26] The unexpected expansion of parenthood was disconcerting for parents, not only because they could not attend to other important matters, but also because it contributed to their growing perceptions that life was no longer "normal," no longer predictable. In sum, the disruption of time-order played a key role in the experiences of disconnection and loss I later discuss.

4 • STIGMA AND DISRUPTED RELATIONSHIPS

Judy is in her early sixties, but you would not know it. Slim and energetic with short hair that is neatly cut, I would have taken her for a younger woman. Classical music was playing in her living room when she welcomed me into her home, and we sat comfortably on the couch while she told me about her son. Jason, who is now twenty-five years old, was diagnosed with ADHD when he was in elementary school. Judy says that while he is "adventuresome" and "a natural athlete," his learning disability has prevented him from making much of his life so far. His grades were mediocre throughout junior high and high school, and after failing out of college during his freshman year at a university, his mom says he is "on the ten-year plan" at a nearby state school.

Grades were not Jason's only problem while he was still living at home. He was prone to disobeying his parents, drank alcohol, smoked marijuana, and occasionally threatened to run away. Judy says that other parents sometimes saw Jason as a "problem child." One Fourth of July when Jason was in his mid-teens, for example, he invited a group of friends over to spend the night, and they decided to build a firecracker. The boys filled some clear plastic tubing with the flash powder from store-bought firecrackers, attached a makeshift fuse, and tried to ignite it. To their disappointment, they could not get the homemade firecracker to explode, so they gave up and left the device at the end of Jason's driveway. When Judy returned from running some errands the next morning, a police car was parked at the end of her street, preventing traffic from entering her cul-de-sac. Apparently, a neighbor had seen the firecracker, thought it was a bomb, and called the police.

Having stayed over the night before, Jason's friends were still at his house, and the police officers insisted on talking to them. In the end, the officers did not bring charges against the boys because it was clear that they had not intended to harm anyone. Nonetheless, Judy and her husband, Tom, later contacted the other children's parents to discuss what had happened. As it turned out, one of the mothers was furious. Judy said,

> We knocked on the door, and we just wanted to let them know that everything was gonna be okay. If you could have seen the look on the other mother's face when she saw it was us at the door! She was angry. She was hostile. And I wasn't ready for that. I *knew* her. She wasn't my closest friend, but I knew her well enough. My face got red. I could feel my face flush. I cannot convey to you what the feeling was. . . . When you get to be a certain age . . . you've experienced all the embarrassment of life . . . but this time I was caught off guard, and I just was not expecting her reaction at all.

Judy and Tom tried their best to mend the situation, and they made Jason apologize to his friend's parents. But despite their efforts, the mother and father requested that Jason not spend any more time with their son. Judy explained,

> Jason was very disrespectful toward [my husband] and me when he was at their house. . . . I'm sure that [the other parents] thought . . . "This is inexcusable . . . Why don't they control this child?" . . . I mean, they didn't understand the ADD aspects of this. They just saw parents who obviously weren't in control of their child. . . . I was concerned about seeing [them] the next time. I really was.

This chapter explores how children's problems disrupted parents' relationships with acquaintances, friends, and family members, as well as with one another. Stigma, though not the only mechanism of disruption, often served to disconnect parents from their ordinary social circles. Not all of the parents I interviewed were like Judy, with children who misbehaved or were "delinquent" per se. However, all had children who violated people's expectations. Stigma has the tendency to "spread from the stigmatized individual to his [or her] close connections."[1] Indeed, parents sometimes experienced "courtesy stigma" because of their close connection to stigmatized children. However, as Judy's story illustrates, stigma was sometimes a matter of parent-blame. When people held parents accountable for causing or failing to control children's problems, parents were stigmatized not because of mere association, but because people perceived them to be "bad parents." Previous research has not differentiated between courtesy stigma and the stigma of bad parenting. As I illustrate, this distinction is not only more empirically accurate, but it also helps us to understand why stigma affected some groups of parents more than others.

Although stigma was, perhaps, the most salient dimension of parents' relationship troubles, the disruption of routine and disagreements about the nature and appropriate treatment of children's "problems" also played a role. Like all relationships, parents' marriages, friendships, and kinships were embedded in social order. No longer held securely intact by shared definitions of the situation and the temporal order of daily life, these relationships were no longer easy, taken-for-granted features of parents' personal worlds. As they changed in response to other forms of disruption, relationships themselves became sites and sources of family trouble.[2]

RELATIONSHIPS AND THE DISRUPTION OF ROUTINE

Just as the expansion of parenthood diminished parents' ability to take care of themselves, it left them little time for building and sustaining relationships. In the previous chapter, for example, I quoted Sam, who said that his seventeen-year-old daughter's attention deficit disorder (diagnosed in the sixth-grade) had become the household's primary focus. Reflecting on how his daily life had been affected by his daughter's problems in school, he remarked, "I see [my daughter's problems] as probably having limited me from expressing myself in other ways, [from] doing some things that I don't have time for now . . . socializing with people, friends . . . I think it has shortened our social circle." As Sam's comment illustrates, spending time with friends was yet another part of parents' lives that was put on hold when children's "problems" emerged. Several mothers said that tending to their children's problems meant that they gave less attention to those children's siblings. This, too, was a common source of regret. Claire, whose nine-year-old son was diagnosed with autism when he was three, said that although she feels very little guilt about her younger son's autism, she does feel bad about giving him such a disproportionate amount of her time and energy.

> I feel a little bit of guilt about [my older son]. . . . I mean, you can only give so much, you know? . . . We went on this trip, and I remembered [our younger son's] medication, but I hadn't remembered [our older son's]. And so I go to get the [insurance] card, [and I've] got two of [our younger son's cards] and none of [our older son's]. And I thought, "You know, this is just emblematic. I give so much to [my younger son]." And in school I just expect [his brother] to take care of himself, you know?

The lack of time for investing in other relationships was particularly hard on some parents' marriages. Eve and Tim's seventeen-year-old son has Fragile X syndrome, and signs of his condition had emerged when he was a toddler. Eve described how her son's disabilities changed her and Tim's relationship.

I think a couple's intimate life . . . it diminishes. You don't have that spontaneity time, you don't have that intimate time. You don't have what other typical
families would have. . . . Sexually it's very difficult because you're on all the time
and it's difficult to tell your special needs child, "I'm sorry we need to have this
privacy." . . . We went, one time, two years without ever going out to dinner by
ourselves. I mean, never even ever getting a burger by ourselves for two years. . . .
There are aspects of your relationship that get put on hold.

Even when parents did find time to spend with one another, they often were
so worn thin from worry and exhaustion that their time spent together was not
as enjoyable or connecting as it used to be. Peter's six-year-old son has trouble
controlling his emotions and is aggressive with other children. These problems
first manifested when he was four years old. Peter explained,

Even after the boys were asleep at night, [we were] too worn out from it to do
anything other than just to go to bed or, you know, watch a movie and just kind
of be catatonic for a while. So yeah, it had an effect [on our relationship]. I mean,
luckily, I think, it's a strong enough relationship that . . . it never became a source
of tension or conflict that kind of split us apart.

Also troubling for parents' marriages were disagreements about the household division of labor. This, too, stemmed from the expansion of parenthood
and lack of time; some mothers resented the extra carework related to children's
problems and wanted their spouses to shoulder more responsibility. For example, Kathy, whose six-year-old son was diagnosed with cerebral palsy before his
first birthday, expressed frustration at her husband's reluctance to take their son
to doctor's appointments.

It was always on me to deal with [our son]. . . . That was hard for me at first, and
it caused tensions within our marriage. . . . The agreement was that I would do
all the appointments and stay at home with [our son], and then [my husband]
would work as much he could to cover for everything. Which was fine the first
year. But after that, when I decided that my mom could take care of [our son] . . .
I went back to work. I was probably off for about a year and a half. And then I was
like, "Okay." You know? "Now you can start helping with the appointments." But
he just [resisted].

Given how much stress parents were already under, even small disagreements
about the division of carework could escalate quickly. Jessica recalled a recent
argument with Peter.

I'm not having any time with my younger son . . . and so I said that [to Peter]. And he said, you know, "Well, it's too bad that I couldn't do it," you know, "my job doesn't let me do it" . . . and I probably interpreted it wrong. . . . I probably interpreted it like, "Well, you know, if only I had time, I'd do it," kind of thing (laughs). . . . But that's the thing, you know, after you get stressed, your defenses wear down, and you're more likely to react. Overreact to things, you know? So I just . . . argh! I just got mad when he said that, "if only he could do it." [I thought], "Well, you see how easy it is! I wish you could do it!"

While the disruption of routine was one means by which children's problems troubled parents' marriages, the challenges posed by increased carework and diminished time and energy were nothing compared to those stemming from disagreements about how to define and treat children's conduct. When discussing her husband's reluctance to attend doctor's appointments, for example, Kathy added, "I think some of it was just [that my husband] couldn't accept [our son's condition] completely either." Like Kathy, a number of women said that their husband's lack of participation was a symptom of their "denial," which was, for them, a much more serious problem.

DISAGREEMENTS ABOUT THE NATURE AND TREATMENT OF CHILDREN'S PROBLEMS

Intimate partnerships are important venues for reality maintenance where people continuously develop and verify taken-for-granted ideas about themselves and the world around them.[3] This existential "function" of intimate relationships is such that separation, divorce, and death often trouble people's identities and worldviews.[4] Interviews with parents demonstrate how the opposite also holds true: when something undermines a couple's taken-for-granted understanding of reality, the relationship itself can become vulnerable.

Children's problems challenged a number of parents' working assumptions about their children and childrearing. Now uncertain about who their children were, who they would become, how they would develop or behave, and how they would respond to remedial efforts, parents were also unsure about how they should parent. "The question as to what it is that is going on"[5] was no longer readily available. The uncertainty that characterized children's "problems" provided fertile ground for definitional disagreements between parents, as I discussed in previous chapters. These arguments disrupted participants' marriages in serious ways. A common dynamic was for fathers to become increasingly distant or paralyzed at the same time that mothers were becoming increasingly frenetic in their efforts to solve what they saw as "the problem." Andrea's nineteen-year-old daughter has had drug and alcohol problems since the tenth-grade. She was diagnosed with depression in junior high school and has also been in trouble for fighting. Andrea explained how her daughter's depression and substance abuse was a catalyst for marital trouble.

> I really was a crazy woman then, I think. I mean, now looking back at it. And it put a huge strain on my husband's and my relationship. Because I was the one obsessing. And he was the one that was just beside himself, not knowing what to do, but felt that I was not doing the right thing. And I was resentful that he was feeling I wasn't doing the right thing . . . when you have a crisis like this, it really brings out your different approaches . . . we went to family counseling ourselves.

Fathers were less likely than mothers to discuss marital conflict, but when they did talk about how children's problems affected their marriages, their accounts of the situation tended to align with mothers' accounts. This might have been because, among the couples that stayed together, men eventually adopted their spouses' points of view. Sergio and Joan's fifteen-year-old son began showing symptoms of mental illness when he was eleven, and doctors think he may develop schizophrenia. Sergio and Joan were on the brink of separation when Joan encouraged Sergio to see a therapist. They also sought couples counseling. By the time I interviewed Sergio, he, like Joan, framed his previous definitions of the situation as "denial." He said,

> There was tension between us. Because she is the type that will do the research, that will spend until three o'clock in the morning on the computer researching and researching and researching. . . . My focus was just to keep the family together and pay the bills. . . . It probably took another six months before I fully got on board with the research. . . . I [had] that mentality of, "Oh, he'll grow out of it. He's just having a bad day, just snap out of it." You know, and [my wife would say], "You don't know what you're talking about." I was in denial. And then my therapist opened my eyes.

I spoke with two divorced couples, and, in those cases, one father concurred with his ex-spouse's definition of the child's "problems" and the other did not. Jason, whose six-year-old son was diagnosed with autism when he was eighteen months old, thought that his ex-wife's efforts on behalf of their son were entirely warranted. He explained,

> She threw herself into it whole-heartedly and given the circumstances, I felt like I was supportive of that. . . . We've had our differences, but it really did not revolve around anything she's been doing on [our son's] behalf. You know, she read a lot. She did a lot of the research . . . put him on the special diet pretty

early on and saw results. . . . She kept me in the loop enough to understand the challenges that were ahead and what needed to be done to work the system to get the services we needed.

Craig, in contrast, fundamentally disagreed with his ex-wife's definition of the situation. Craig's sixteen-year-old daughter has had academic and behavioral problems since sixth-grade. She has experimented with self-cutting, attempted suicide, and is on anti-depressant medication. Craig explained,

> [My ex-wife] decided that [our daughter] was mentally ill. . . . Nowadays, I mean, there's something wrong with you, abnormal about you, if you're not on some sort of pill, I think. You know, it's like, what was the joke? Why don't you go take a Valium like a normal person or something? So it's so easy to get this stuff.

Unresolved disagreements about children's "problems" were probably common among parents who were separated or divorced. Though I did not interview most ex-husbands or estranged spouses, a handful of mothers said that definitional conflicts contributed to the dissolution of their marriages. Amanda's son was fifteen years old at the time of the interview and, in the past ten years, has been diagnosed with attention deficit/hyperactivity disorder, dyslexia, and bipolar disorder. Amanda said that her ex-husband's denial about their son's "problems" contributed to their separation. She said:

> I think that [our son's] situation brought out part of my ex-husband's personality that I don't think I really recognized when we were first together . . . [he's] not sensitive to illness at all and his insensitivity to his children on that level . . . I definitely think it was part of [why we separated].

It was not just parents' marriages that were beset by disagreements over the nature and appropriate handling of children's "problems." Parents' relationships with friends and family members faced similar challenges. However, unlike the disagreements between mothers and fathers—which tended to focus on whether or not a "problem" existed or how much work was necessary to remedy "the problem"—conflicts between parents, family members, and friends more commonly centered on "the problem's" ostensible cause. In these cases, the stigma of being a "bad parent" underpinned relationship disruption.

COURTESY STIGMA AND THE STIGMA OF BAD PARENTING

Social psychologists use Goffman's concept of courtesy stigma[6] to examine the accounts of parents whose children have disabilities.[7] Their research illustrates how caring for a child with disabilities alters one's place in the prevailing social order, undermines claims to "normalcy," and disrupts valued relationships and identities. The stigma can be felt or enacted—parents sometimes experience isolation and shame because they anticipate negative labeling, while, in other cases, rejection and discrimination are directly manifest in interaction.[8] In any case, courtesy stigma adds to the subjective burden of caring for a disabled child[9] and is linked to mental health problems, such as depression.[10]

In some cases, parents experienced courtesy stigma just as Goffman defined it. Carol, for example, said that she does not see her own parents or siblings very often and wishes that she had more support from her extended family. She suspects they are reluctant to visit because they are uncomfortable with her son's Asperger's syndrome. She said, "I think it may be very scary for [my parents and siblings], very uncomfortable. It's, 'Oh, we have an autistic child in the family, I don't know what to do, I don't know how I'm gonna handle this.' You know, they've never said that, but I kind of wonder about that sometimes." Carol's thirteen-year-old son was diagnosed with Asperger's syndrome when he was four. As her comment demonstrates, by distancing themselves from children who were "different," people also withdrew from those children's mothers and fathers. Sergio's fifteen-year-old son began showing symptoms of mental illness when he was eleven. Doctors think he may develop schizophrenia. Sergio recalled how his son's problems diminished the family's social network.

> [Nathan] is quiet. He's different. He has long hair, plays guitar, he dresses up with punk clothing. . . . We went to a barbeque with a bunch of kids who were out there playing baseball, they were really athletic. And they were all, "Come on, [Nathan], let's go play baseball, let's go play football!" And the other parents are going, "What's wrong with [Nathan]? How come [he] isn't out there playing sports?" . . . It got to the point now to where we don't get invited a lot.

While friends and family members sometimes kept their distance, some parents said that they actively retreated from their previous social circles. Patty's thirteen-year-old son was diagnosed with autism when he was fifteen months old. Patty's husband had become a stay-at-home father in order to help administer their autistic son's home program. As Patty explained, the differences between their lives and the lives of "normal" families make socializing with other parents unbearable.

> It's too hard . . . because their lives are so different. . . . It's in your face, seeing how different your life is. . . . So there's always, I guess, how do I say it? Failures. Lots of failures that you're reminded of. . . . It is [painful] because they can easily do things that we can't easily do, or sometimes they'll be talking about their jobs.

Well, I can talk about [my job], but then [my husband] can't talk about his. So yeah, we don't socialize as a couple at all outside of our family.

The previous comments evince courtesy stigma; in these particular cases, parents felt estranged from particular family members or friends not because of attributes that they themselves possessed, but because their identities and daily lives were tightly bound to stigmatized children. In other words, stigma stemmed from *close social proximity* to discredited others. In other cases, however, stigma was not just a matter of social proximity, but also a matter of *assumed culpability*. When people held them accountable for causing or failing to remedy children's problems, parents experienced the stigma of being "bad parents." Anna's mother, for example, was so embarrassed by her granddaughter's developmental delays that she asked Anna not to come to a relative's wedding. She told Anna quite directly that she thought "the problem" was poor parenting. "My mom actually had a very hard time accepting my daughter's special needs," Anna recalled, "and thought it was bad parenting . . . [she] was saying, 'What? You're not training her right.'" Mothers commonly said that the intimation of blame prevented them from forming relationships with other parents. Maria, whose son was identified as gifted but had gotten into trouble for misbehaving and starting fights, said,

[People] always saw my son as the problem child in class. And I think their tendency is to blame the parent. . . . I haven't really formed any relationships with parents of my son's peers. . . . There was a new parent one year, her daughter was new to the school . . . and I talked to her, like one of the first days of school. And she's really nice and open and talkative. And then a couple weeks into, when she really—in my perception—found out who I was the parent of, well then suddenly . . . I felt a difference.

For reasons I explain later, mothers experienced the stigma of bad parenting more frequently and saliently than fathers did. However, fathers were not immune to blame. Phil's seventeen-year-old son began using and selling drugs three years ago. He was diagnosed with ADHD when he was in the sixth-grade and has also been in trouble for fighting. Phil was concerned about how other parents would perceive him when his son returned from a therapeutic boarding school. He explained,

One of the things we've talked about doing when he comes home this week is going to a basketball game [at his high school]. . . . That will be very uncomfortable for me, frankly. Because a lot of those parents I've had no contact with [since my son left for recovery]. I'm not looking forward to it at all. Frankly, [my wife and I have] been on the other end. And I know what I've thought. I'm not a cruel person, but . . . I'd say, "Something is wrong there . . . something the parents did." And now I'm sort of on the reverse end of it. And I don't blame anybody for look- ing necessarily cross-eyed at us or making judgments. . . . . Going to the game, they're all gonna be there in one place, and you open yourself up to gossip and all the other kind of stuff.

Although previous research acknowledges blame as part of the stigma that parents experience when children have problems, scholars have not clearly distinguished between courtesy stigma and the stigma of bad parenting. As illustrated here, this distinction is conceptually important. When parents are stigmatized because of ostensible culpability for children's problems, their iden- tities are tainted not by mere association but because they are the direct tar- gets of moral judgment. This is not a straightforward manifestation of courtesy stigma and is more appropriately analyzed as a dual stigma premised on close social proximity *and* assumed culpability. The distinction is also more empiri- cally accurate. Some participants experienced courtesy stigma in the absence of blame. Others experienced blame occasionally, but it was not a salient feature of their stories. Still others placed blame at the center of their accounts. Among the parents I interviewed, mothers, the parents of children with invisible disabilities, and the parents of young children were far more susceptible to blame than other groups of parents were. It appeared that parents' experiences of stigmatization were shaped by gendered constructions of parenthood, assumptions about what constitutes a legitimate disability, and notions about young children's innocence and fragility.

GENDERED CONSTRUCTIONS OF PARENTHOOD

Due to their greater social proximity and ostensible culpability for children's problems, women were more likely than men to experience both courtesy stigma and blame. Jessica's six-year-old son has trouble controlling his emotions and is aggressive with other children. These problems first manifested when he was four years old. Jessica talked at length about stigma and was particularly focused on the experience of blame.

I imagine [people] think that my parenting is poor, I'm not setting enough limits, the kid is getting away with things he shouldn't, he's spoiled. . . . [Two parents] wanted to have [our son] kicked out of the [preschool] program because of his behavior. And every time I see [one of them] in town, I just get these emotions.

As a stay-at-home mother, Jessica is in close contact with her son throughout the day. Because she volunteers regularly at his preschool, she is also in frequent contact with teachers and other parents. In contrast, her husband, Peter, works outside of the home. Although he performs routine childcare in the evenings and on weekends, his daily activities are not tightly bound to those of his son. Peter's account was markedly different from Jessica's. When interviewed separately, he said the following: "There were a couple of times when [our son], either with another child in preschool or with an adult there, became physically violent. And I think some of the other parents were frustrated with that and concerned for their children. Maybe irritated. . . . You know, I wasn't there for it. But it came to a point when there was actually a request that [he] leave the preschool." While Jessica's account provides a clear-cut example of dual stigma, Peter's comments evince neither courtesy stigma nor parent-blame. The difference stems, in part, from these parents' relative social proximity to the stigmatized child. Because she has spent time at the school, Jessica is familiar with the parents who attempted to have her son expelled. As she indicates, stigma is enacted when she encounters those parents in public. Peter, on the other hand, "wasn't there for it." He knows of the situation, but his recollections are second hand, and stigma is not a salient feature of his experiences.

Approximately half of the women I interviewed were stay-at-home mothers, and, in all but three cases, women who worked outside of the home still performed a majority of routine childcare. Accompanying children to playgrounds, grocery stores, doctor's offices, and other public venues meant that mothers encountered courtesy stigma and blame more frequently than fathers did. Parents' interviews also suggest that women's friendships were more closely tied (or socially proximal) to children and childrearing. As this comment from Jessica illustrates, stigma often was disruptive to women's social connections: "It does affect my social life. I'm sure I would get together with more parents for play dates and things . . . [but] I always have to think about that stress . . . how will [my son] behave? Is he gonna behave okay? Am I gonna have to leave the park? Leave the house? Sometimes I just don't wanna deal with that. So I think I've become a bit isolated." Comments like these were less common among fathers. Here is how Peter responded when asked if his son's problems had impacted his social life: "I've got a pretty demanding job, so to be honest, I don't have a lot of friendships outside of that. I mean, we have a few family friends, I've got my brother and my family and a couple of people I get together with occasionally or catch up with over lunch or whatever. But my personal network is a pretty small one. A lot of my social interaction is through my work. . . ." From Peter's perspective, his work outside of the home precludes an extensive personal network. His job is his primary venue for social interaction, and those interactions are not predicated upon or directly connected to his son. Consequently, there are fewer opportunities for his son's troubles to disrupt those interactions.

While women's close social proximity to children is taken for granted, feminist scholars point out that routine childcare is a political matter. Indeed, proximity is not a "given" phenomenon but an outcome of how people construct gender and caregiving. Although the time fathers spend parenting has increased over the last several decades, women still perform a majority of routine childcare.[11] As I discussed in a previous chapter, women's disproportionate participation in children's affairs is tied to an ideology that conceives of childrearing as an essentially feminine enterprise.[12] Contemporary constructions of good mothering (intensive mothering, concerted cultivation) require close physical and social proximity by calling for large investments of women's time and energy.[13] To the extent that child-centered orientations to care encourage mothers to construct social and emotional lives that are predicated upon their children, women are particularly susceptible to stigmatization.

Women also assumed greater culpability for children's conditions and behaviors. Even when fathers did encounter stigma, they were less likely to interpret negative attention as blame. For example, Judy, the mother whose son built the makeshift firecracker, placed blame at the center of her story. She felt discredited because the acquaintance seemed to view her as a bad mother. When I interviewed Tom, Judy's husband, on a separate occasion, he told the same story. However, it was clear that he did not share Judy's interpretation.

TOM: One of the neighbors finally said, "We don't want our kid playing with your son anymore." Well that was devastating, as far as I was concerned.
ARA: When you say devastating . . .
TOM: Ego. Ego! You know, this is our kid, and I was angry at them, the other parents. . . . I don't know if embarrassment is the right word. But it's close. Yeah, there was an ego problem for me. "You don't like my kid?" [I was] disappointed, certainly.

To the extent that Tom faced a challenge to his self-concept ("ego") and experienced negative emotion ("devastation"), his account can be analyzed in terms of courtesy stigma. However, there is nothing in this account that suggests a perception of blame. Tom recounts anger and disappointment, but unlike Judy he does not imagine that others think he is a bad father.

It is likely that mothers are more sensitized to the prospect of blame because they are held disproportionately culpable for children's conduct. Mother-blame reached its heyday in the 1940s and '50s, and, in the decades that followed, mothers became scapegoats for everything from schizophrenia to serial killing. At different times in the last sixty-five years, the public has blamed mothers for autism, homosexuality, youth rebellion, children's poor school performance, low self-esteem, and poverty.[14] This historical context goes a long way toward explaining why the women in the study perceive parent-blame more often than fathers do.

These data further suggest that people were, in fact, more likely to hold mothers culpable for children's problems. Two fathers in this study were their children's primary caregivers, and their accounts illustrate this point. Like the mothers quoted in the previous section, both fathers were in close social proximity to children and both emphasized how children's problems negatively impacted their social lives. The first father, Bill, has a sixteen-year-old son with a seizure disorder and developmental disabilities (conditions that developed in infancy). He commented, "You lose your friends because of having a special needs child. You know, a) they're afraid they're gonna catch it, b) they don't understand it, c) they don't want to deal with it, it's too depressing. They just don't want to be around your child. They don't want to be reminded of how lucky they are." The second father, Daniel, has an eighteen-year-old son with ill-defined learning disabilities. Daniel's son began exhibiting intellectual and social delays when he was four years old, and he has been diagnosed with auditory processing disorder and attention deficit/hyperactivity disorder. Daniel discussed how caring for his son, who still lives at home, has impacted his romantic relationships.

> I've dated a little bit off and on, and [one relationship] was serious . . . [but] she started asking, "What's [it] gonna be like with [your son]? How long is he gonna live with you?" And I said, "See ya." The woman that I am eventually with . . . is gonna have to accept the fact that [my son] might be around for a little longer.

Both of these excerpts indicate courtesy stigma, but neither of these fathers perceived parent-blame. When asked directly about the stigma of being a bad parent, both men said that, on the contrary, people respected and praised their paternal performances.

BILL: Dads have a lot of weight [in educational settings]. . . . You can see how tones change when a dad walks in the room. . . . When dads come on board, it's like everything kind of opens up. . . . When [teachers] know that dad is in the picture and dad is working on the homework . . . it's a win-win.
DANIEL: [I have a] very close-knit family, brothers and sisters and nieces and nephews . . . [they tell me] "Daniel, you're a friggin' saint for doing what you do." . . . I have had a couple guy friends that said, "I couldn't do it." You know, "Give him back to his mom."

While people take women's care work for granted, they celebrate fathers who participate in routine childcare. "A dad who knows the name of his kids' pediatrician and reads them stories at night is a saint; a mother who doesn't is a sinner."[15] As Bill and Dan's accounts suggest, the tendency to idealize involved fathers might result in a halo effect, making it less likely for people to view men as culpable for children's problems, even when those men are in close social proximity to stigmatized children.

These data highlight the political nature of parents' stigmatization; men and women experience stigma differently because dominant constructions of motherhood and fatherhood place men at a relative advantage. Nonetheless, the importance of gender in shaping parents' experiences of stigma should not be overstated. Fathers do sometimes experience both types of stigma, and my data suggest that two additional factors—the type of stigma children carried and the children's ages—play key roles in which parents perceive and encounter blame.

CHILDREN'S STIGMA TYPE AND THE CONSTRUCTION OF DISABILITY

There are three types of stigma: deviant physical attributes, or what Goffman called "abominations of the body"; "blemishes of individual character," related to one's personality, moral standards, or beliefs; and "tribal stigma," or affiliation with a deviant race, religion, or nationality.[16] Deviant attributes do not automatically give rise to one type of stigma or another, and a single attribute can be categorized in different ways, depending on the social context. Medicalization has resulted in a large-scale shift toward viewing deviant attributes in biomedical rather than moral terms.[17] Although medicalization does not eliminate stigma, it does change the nature of assumed culpability because disability and disease accounts have the potential to render individuals less blameworthy.[18] In this context, assumptions about the underlying nature of children's "problems"—and whether or not a child was viewed as having a "legitimate" disability—shaped parents' experiences of stigma.

Parent-blame was rarely a salient feature of parents' accounts when children had clearly discernible, uncontested physical conditions such as severe cerebral palsy. In fact, these mothers and fathers were sometimes validated as good parents precisely because they parented children with special needs. Sarah's thirteen-year-old biological son was diagnosed with cerebral palsy at birth and is severely disabled. Sarah's ex-husband had challenged her need for ongoing child support, and, when the judge ruled in Sarah's favor, she praised the mother's full-time caregiving. Sarah explained:

[The judge] really affirmed me and said, "This mother is doing a great job. . . ." And then she looked at [my ex-husband] and his attorney and said, ". . . You should be glad that you married her and not someone else. You married some-one that will take care of your son."

This is not to suggest that the parents of children with traditional disabilities did not experience guilt; as I discuss in the next chapter, such feelings were common among most of the parents interviewed, especially among mothers. However, parents whose children carried a physical stigma usually emphasized that others did not blame them for having caused children problems. When I asked Jody, whose nineteen-year-old son was diagnosed with cerebral palsy at birth, about blame, here is how she responded: "No, no one has ever blamed me. I've never felt that way at all, unless I go out to a conference or something and I listen to a professional talk about [how] it's so critical [during the] first three months that you're pregnant to see that you don't take any alcohol or [anything] that affects the midline development of the baby . . . but that wasn't intentional to place that upon me." This excerpt illustrates that self-doubt and guilt are not, in all cases, manifestations of stigma. As Jody explains, knowledge of how a mother's behav-ior can influence fetal development gives her pause, but she does not believe that anyone has ever blamed her for her son's disability.

Jody's comments also illustrate how medical accounts simultaneously ame-liorate mother-blame while rendering women accountable for children's condi-tions in other ways. The proliferation of research on fetal development has led to a policing of women's bodies, and maternal self-doubt is pervasive, regardless of whether or not children have discrediting attributes.[19] Medical accounts also can shift culpability away from matters of causation and toward matters of "appro-priate" treatment and care.[20] Lisa, whose nine-year-old son sustained brain dam-age shortly after birth, said the following when I asked her about blame: "Um . . . [I've felt blamed] somewhat by my in-laws, that's sad to say. . . . [My mother-in-law] is like, 'Why can't you potty train him?' You know, and I have felt that pres-sure . . . but by society? Not so much so." In Lisa's perception, her in-laws do not implicate her as the source of her son's disabilities, but they do view her as failing to "normalize" his conduct. This renders her susceptible to parent-blame, despite her son's physical stigma. Nonetheless, we must take seriously Lisa's comment that she does not feel blamed "by society." This statement suggests that, despite interactions with her mother-in-law, she does not believe that people *in general* blame her for her son's problems.

Accounts like these stood in contrast to the comments of men and women whose children's problems were viewed in terms of "moral failure." Among these parents were the mothers and fathers of teenaged and adult children who abused alcohol and drugs, ran away, had trouble with the law, or could not maintain jobs or romantic relationships. When I interviewed Seth, his nineteen-year-old daughter was sober and living at home. However, Seth remembered what it was like when she was fourteen, had run away, and was living on the streets:

We're bad parents! I mean, otherwise, why would your kid run away? . . . How do you tell your friends what your kid is doing? . . . I knew that there were a lot of people making all kinds of . . . little judgments about who I was and what I've done and why I was a bad parent.

Unlike participants whose children carried a physical stigma, parents like Seth took for granted that others blamed them for children's problems. Efforts to medicalize substance addiction have been only partially successful, and the problems displayed by these teens are broadly understood as matters of character.[21] These data suggest that perceived moral lapses serve to discredit parents directly, with more frequency and greater salience than physical forms of deviance.

It is important to note, however, that parent-blame in such cases was often mitigated by children's own ostensible culpability. Parents whose teenaged and adult children carried character stigmas often framed deviant conduct as a "choice." Later in the interview, Seth commented, "We're trying to be these great new age parents, helping our kid out, giving her all these choices, and she's choosing shit, you know? Why is she doing that? I mean, she could have anything! And she's doing this!" Deborah, whose twenty-six-year-old son has been an alcoholic since he was fifteen, made a similar comment. "You always have a certain sense of 'I could have done better' when you're a parent," she explained, "but I really didn't take on the responsibility of [my son's] choices. . . . He knew how I felt about drinking in general. . . . I don't think I felt like I had caused it, you know?" As these quotes demonstrate, parents' sense of culpability was somewhat reduced when children were viewed as responsible for their own problems. Perceptions about agency and substance abuse appeared to curtail the stigma of bad parenting among this group of mothers and fathers.

It was among parents whose children had invisible disabilities—mild autism or Asperger's syndrome, attention deficit disorder, learning disabilities, and inconspicuous mental health problems and developmental delays—that parent-blame was paramount. While parents (and especially mothers) framed such "problems" in biomedical terms, strangers, friends, family members, teachers, and school administrators often viewed children's "problems" as matters of character. Previous research suggests that conditions that are ostensibly biological but not discernible to the everyday observer are particularly stigmatizing for parents.[22] When children look "normal," people expect them to behave accordingly, and they interpret deviance as a "problem" of character for which parents are responsible.

Medical accounts could not be wielded in all cases to mitigate the stigma of bad parenting. When parent-blame was enacted in interactions with strangers, for example, the parents of children with invisible disabilities usually found it untenable to correct others' assumptions about the nature of children's "problems."[23] Olivia and Jerry, whose ten-year-old adopted son has learning and behavioral problems caused by a brain injury sustained at birth, had the following exchange.

OLIVIA: I always want to say, "Brain damage!" You know? (Laughs).
JERRY: Yeah. He's not spoiled, he's brain-damaged.
OLIVIA: He has brain damage! [...] I try to be cool, but it's kind of tough.... I [don't] want to say in front of [my son], "He's brain damaged," or "he's disabled"... [so] I ignore them or tell them to mind their own business or whatever.

Parents sensed that, even if it were to reduce their own culpability, overtly framing children's "problems" in biomedical terms risked greater stigmatization for children. Among strangers, then, this group of participants rarely attempted to ameliorate the negative effects of parent-blame.

In the contemporary United States, biomedical accounts carry a social premium because they have the potential to reduce culpability and the negative effects of stigma. As these data illustrate, parents' experiences of stigma reflected popular distinctions between disability and deviance. The former categorization served to diminish the stigma of bad parenting, while the latter encouraged it. However, what constitutes a disability is contested, and it was when people disagreed about the nature of children's "problems" that parents were most susceptible to the bad parent label.

CHILDREN'S AGES AND THE CONSTRUCTION OF INNOCENCE

Parenthood embeds people in particular social networks, strengthening some relationships and weakening others. People with children have more contact with neighbors,[24] their relationships with extended kin and non-kin are more likely to involve caregiving,[25] and women with children are encouraged to befriend other mothers.[26] Parents' accounts suggest that this close connection between the social worlds of parents and children renders men and women particularly vulnerable to courtesy stigma when *young* children are discredited. First, mothers and fathers spend more time engaged in childcare activities when children are young.[27] This also is the period that parents usually begin to form relationships with other parents. Parents whose children carried stigma at a young age said that they had few opportunities to develop such friendships, and they became increasingly isolated. Tim's son, now seventeen years old, has a genetic disorder and cognitive disabilities. Tim became aware of his son's condition when he just a toddler. This father explained,

> People are often uncomfortable with someone who is different from them. And so you see this kid making all these weird noises, these weird facial expressions, things like this. And people were just uncomfortable with it. . . . Friends that had kids [our son's] age . . . those kids wanted to hang out with other "normal" kids, if I may use that term . . . so as the time went on, our world became more and more insulated.

While parents whose children developed problems as teenagers did experience dual stigma in the context of their personal relationships, they were less likely to report that these experiences resulted in isolation. In fact, they commonly described friends and acquaintances as understanding and supportive, despite moments of awkwardness or perceived blame. Unlike the parents of young children, many of these participants had well-developed and long-standing friendships with other parents before children developed problems, and they used these relationships as sources of support. Steve and Marie discovered six months ago that their seventeen-year-old daughter is a cocaine addict. Steve described how he and his wife drew strength from their social networks when their daughter was in a rehabilitation facility.

> We've been in town for twenty years. [My wife] has been very active in the time we've been here . . . and has made some wonderful friends over the years. She drew on those experiences, and she called [other parents] and said, "You may or may not have heard this . . . [our daughter] is in a [psychiatric] facility, and we're contemplating our options." . . . Support is good. There's strength in numbers.

As this quote suggests, stigma resulted in less isolation among parents whose children developed problems as teenagers and young adults. Once parents established relationships with other parents, those relationships were less predicated upon children's conduct—or *less proximal* to children's affairs—and children's stigmatizing conditions were less likely to disrupt those relationships.

Youth also appeared to increase the likelihood of parent-blame. Unless children had traditional disabilities, they were assumed to have greater control over their conduct as they grew older. Age—coupled with stigma type—shaped assumptions about children's culpability. This is particularly evident in the way parents' narratives about the "problems" changed over time. In several cases, conditions labeled as invisible "disabilities" among young children were re-narrated as "problems" of character among teenaged and adult children. For example, Andrea described her daughter as suffering from depression in junior high school: "In the seventh grade she had a period of depression . . . she did some cutting, some minor cutting on her wrists. And that was the sort of the sentinel thing that made me realize that she needed more help than I was able to provide. So we did get her into counseling . . . she had a mental health evaluation. . . . I kinda just assumed, 'She's gonna need some help.'" Her daughter (now nineteen years old) continued to have problems in high school, and, by the time I interviewed Andrea, she framed her daughter's "problems" largely in terms of substance abuse and poor choices.

> When she turned eighteen, we said, "You know, this is it. There's no more. You are on your own with whatever happens. If you get in trouble, you must pay your own consequences. . . ." I know she is drinking and she is smoking pot still because the boyfriend that she picked still does that. . . . She's no longer working . . . her boyfriend gets into fights. He was arrested for domestic violence, and then she was arrested for domestic violence. . . . My husband and I feel that we can be sympathetic, but . . . you know, she's got to work out her problems. We're not bending over backwards to help her.

These quotes indicate a shift in Andrea's understanding of her daughter's "problems"; while she previously viewed her daughter as having a mental health condition deserving of help, she now believes her daughter must face the consequences of her problems and "work out" things on her own. This shift was evident in a number of cases. It was particularly common for attention deficit disorder to be reframed in terms of character flaws, such as "laziness," as children grew older.

Dominant cultural assumptions about children's fragility and innocence are the heart of the dynamics of culpability described here. In the contemporary United States, the public constructs young children as essentially "good" but infinitely vulnerable and lacking in agency.[28] Intensive parenting models are premised upon children's fragility and the constant dangers they face. To the degree that children cannot be held responsible for poor behavior, people are likely to view parents as culpable for children's problems. As children age, however, they assume greater responsibility for their own conduct, and this appeared to mitigate the stigma of bad parenting.

The disruption of parents' relationships, sometimes through stigma, sometimes through the disruption of routines and taken-for-granted meanings, highlights how trouble materialized and worsened by affecting multiple, foundational aspects of parents' daily lives. Stigma encouraged parents—especially mothers, the parents of children with ill-defined or "invisible" problems, and the parents of young children—to define their situations as troublesome and engage in reme-dial efforts. The disruption caused by remedial efforts further disrupted parents' personal relationships, further compounding their sense that things were "not normal." The more parents felt as though their situations were deeply troubled, the more salient their experiences of stigma were, and so on. Because partici-pants' inner worlds had been connected to and sustained by these now-disrupted social patterns, trouble not only rippled outward into multiple spheres of par-ents' daily lives, but it also spilled inward and churned their emotional worlds. As I discuss in the next two chapters, the forms of disruption described thus far had profound consequences for parents' narratives of self, worldviews, and fun-damental sense of "okay-ness."

5 · UNMET EXPECTATIONS AND EMOTIONAL TURMOIL

Tim and Eve greeted me warmly in the entryway of their home early on a Saturday morning. I had interviewed Eve several months before, so once Tim and I settled in at the kitchen table, she went to a different part of the house to spend time with their seventeen-year-old son, James. I introduced Tim to my research and asked for his consent to participate. Then I asked him to tell me his story. "Start from the beginning," I said, even though my conversation with Eve had given me many of the details.

By the time James was two, his parents were concerned that something might be wrong. He had been slow to meet developmental milestones, but their pediatrician assured them that he was within the range of "normal." They persisted, waiting a long time for an appointment with a sought-after psychiatrist, and that practitioner agreed that *something*, "some type of a major nervous system disorder," was delaying James's development. But there was no clear diagnosis or prognosis. Then, Eve received a phone call from a family member, an aunt whose middle-aged son was developmentally disabled. Recent testing had revealed that the genetic disorder Fragile X syndrome was the source of her son's life-long challenges. Eve, as a blood relative, was possibly a "silent carrier" of the gene mutation. Tim and Eve were not particularly concerned at first; James's development seemed slow, but he did not appear to them to have a serious genetic condition. They requested the test just to be sure, but their doctor was similarly dubious. The results came back positive. Tim thought back to the moment of his son's diagnosis, fifteen years prior to our meeting.

It was really bizarre from a parental standpoint because [the doctor] went from this position of "No, no, no, he doesn't have it," to once the tests came back it was, "Well, you know, you better not expect much out of this kid." I mean, it was just almost like this doomsday scenario. The thing I remember the most about that moment is my wife and I crying and [our son] was just playing in the room. I mean, he had no idea that these people were pronouncing that his chances of making it in life were essentially over. He was just playing at being a kid. And I remember thinking, "All I want to do is go home. I just want to go home. I just want to be in my own house with my own family." It was so hard to digest that absolute bombshell of news, you know? It burns your life to the ground in a figurative sense.

In the months and years that followed, the differences between James and other children became increasingly apparent, and Tim and Eve's lives came to evince the patterns of disruption described in previous chapters. James had high levels of anxiety and was sensitive to sound, so it was difficult to take him to public places. In Tim's words, his son made "weird noises" and "weird facial expressions" that made family members and friends uncomfortable. By the time James was eight or nine, Eve said, most of their friends had "sloughed off," and she and Tim had few connections beyond their family lives. Tim's career plateaued because he and Eve were unwilling to move James out of his familiar environment. Eve decided to become a stay-at-home mother rather than returning to the workforce, as she had previously intended.

Tim and Eve describe themselves as having had different reactions to James's condition and the initial disruption of their routines and relationships during his childhood. In those early years, Eve was simply overwhelmed by day-to-day caretaking. "I'd just sort of muddle through it basically, cry a lot . . . not because of the situation, just because I was just exhausted," she explained. "You still have to go on with your everyday life. I mean it's not like a wound [that] heals and you go on. Everyday you just get up and you just do what you have to do." Tim agreed that working outside the home granted him some degree of emotional distance. "I had some type of a life," he said, "but [Eve] really didn't. Her life was totally and wholly devoted to keeping the house, you know, making sure the bills were paid, and taking care of [James] . . . as hard as it was on me, it had to have been a lot harder on her."

Even so, loss and sorrow were pivotal motifs in Tim's narrative. He described at length the son he and Eve expected to have and his grief at the loss of that imagined child.

[We felt] cheated out of what type of relationship we would have had with [our son] as he would be growing up and, you know, bringing girlfriends home or playing on the football team or playing the oboe in the school concert or whatever, whatever he would have done. Whatever path or trajectory he would have pursued as a child. And as an elementary school kid and as a teenager. We were gonna miss out on all of that. You know, we were never gonna have the bumper sticker on our car saying, "My kid is an honor student at George W. Bush Elementary, or something." So yeah, there were times I think we were both just angry. And angry at life and angry at the world, and angry at our isolation.

You know, I've heard some people say, "Well, you know, we had kids because we want somebody to take care of us when we get old." It never would enter my mind. What a ridiculous reason to have kids! I just kind of thought that, as he grew up, you know, we might find some things in common. Like, whether it was watching football or going on bike rides or playing softball or going on nature walks, watching him play in a high school basketball game, whatever. All those things you just kind of assume are going to happen in life.

And you know, it's interesting. You get married and you have a child, and you just kind of assume all these things about what that's going to be like. You know, your wife is pregnant, and everything seems fine. . . . He's born and he's got, you know, ten fingers and ten toes, and you think everything is great. And then suddenly you find out it's not . . . and it still . . . it hurts. It's not quite the sharp driving pain it was in the earlier days, but you never really get used to it.

In this chapter, I delve into mothers' and fathers' internal worlds, focusing on the emotional dimensions of their troubles. As Tim's words so clearly demonstrate, the "normal child" of parents' imaginations—the child who plays instruments or participates in sports, the child with whom they have something in common—had been a main character in parents' own biographical narratives. That, coupled with the intimacy of parent–child relationships in our contemporary social context, meant that parents' grief for the loss of their children's "normalcy" was profound. What's more, the uncertainty and stigma described in previous chapters fueled strong feelings of anxiety, self-doubt, and guilt. Parents' emotional turmoil, I argue, was yet another factor in the amplification of trouble because suffering was a further catalyst for the disruption of daily routines and relationships.

As Tim indicates when he recalls how James's condition must have been harder on Eve, parents tended to frame mothers as disproportionately affected by children's problems. Scholarship on parenthood, gender, and lived experience might lead us to think that an ideology of intensive motherhood explains this pattern, but my analysis suggests that gendered parenting *practices*, in addition to ideologies, yielded different emotional experiences. I also suggest that the literature on intensive parenting focuses too closely on mothers at the expense of fathers; like Tim, many of the men in this study had deep attachments to fatherhood and family life and were devastated by the troubles stemming from children's problems. In fact, the differences between mothers and fathers did not appear to be as stark as parents themselves made them out to be.

Understanding the emotional features of biographical disruption begins with expectations. It is only against the backdrop of what parents thought their children or childrearing would be like that we can render their feelings intelligible. I conceive of parents' expectations as a key social pattern disrupted in the course of their troubles. If the upheaval stemming from children's problems was like an earthquake, with effects moving outward from the epicenter in waves, parents' expectations were ground zero.

EXPECTATIONS AND THE LOSS OF A "NORMAL" CHILD

As discussed in the introduction, "normal" is a category that no one fully occupies. It is true that some children are "unmarked," their conduct essentially "unproblematic" in the eyes of others. However, being unmarked is not the same as being "normal." All children deviate in some way, at some time, from narrowly-defined, dominant cultural expectations about how children "should be." There is simply too much human variation to speak about "normalcy" with any empirical accuracy. As I explained in Chapter 2, what distinguishes children "with serious problems" from those "without" is a matter of attention and labeling, contingent upon historical, macro- and micro-political processes. Furthermore, "normalcy" is a somewhat nebulous entity, its content and boundaries brought into clear view only when something is defined as "not normal."[1] Thus, it was *after* parents came to view their children as having "significant problems" that they became acutely aware of their own expectation of raising what they came to see as "normal children." Kathy, whose six-year-old son was diagnosed with cerebral palsy before his first birthday, explained,

> I always thought, "Oh, I never have expectations." Because people always say you have these expectations of your children, and I always thought, "Oh, I never did. . . . I don't care if they ever," you know, "go to college. . . ." But after having [my son], then I realized, "No, wait, you do think about that stuff." Because I realized that [he] wasn't going to do those things. And that was hard for me.

Parents articulated "normalcy" in surprisingly similar ways, reciting the benchmarks of the ostensibly typical, middle-class American childhood and early adulthood. Friends, extracurricular activities, good grades, and a college education were the taken-for-granted markers of "normal" children. Debbie, whose twenty-six-year-old son had been an alcoholic since he was a teenager, said the following:

> I pictured [having] these kids that were very involved in all their school stuff and were in and out of here with their buddies . . . doing all the normal things,

you know? The football thing, all of that stuff. Good students, go off to college. Get whatever degree in whatever field and live your life accordingly. And that's not what happened. [My son] was *asked* to leave the high school in the middle of his senior year because he would show up on campus [and] just wouldn't go to class. . . . I never pictured that, I'll tell ya. I never pictured that one of my kids would not graduate from high school.

Children's problems forced parents to recognize and re-examine these expectations. Higher education, especially, is a powerful symbol of middle-class respectability in the contemporary United States. Although a significant proportion of young Americans do not go to college, the parents in this study assumed that their children would earn a bachelor's degree as a matter of course. Sam's daughter, now seventeen, was diagnosed with ADHD when she was in the sixth-grade. She struggles with schoolwork and it is unlikely that she will attend a four-year college directly after graduating from high school. When I asked Sam whether or not he thought that attention deficit/hyperactivity disorder would limit her possibilities, he responded,

I absolutely want the best for her. And [these problems] are holding her back. . . . A lot of the dreams that I had for her won't be possible, . . . education and what comes with that. The ability to be able to excel at something that she really feels good about. To be able to do that in such a way that it can be a benefit to others . . . to let her feel real good about who she is and what she's capable of doing. You know, to be able to earn the things I know she likes.

As Sam's comments demonstrate, the expectation of college was bound tightly to visions of middle-class fulfillment and the dream of securing a meaningful vocation and financially comfortable livelihood. These assumptions about "the good life" reflected parents' own social locations and their unquestioned belief that their children would grow up to be middle-class adults.

Marriage, or a long-term intimate partnership that parents approved of, was another benchmark that participants could no longer take for granted. Parents whose children had mental health problems or substance addictions worried that their sons and daughters would end up with the "wrong" kind of mate. Jessica was already concerned about this possibility, even though her son was only six years old. Her son has trouble controlling his emotions and is aggressive with other children. These problems first manifested when he was four years old.

I worry about his relationship with, you know, intimate relationships. He does have trouble connecting emotionally. . . . He's so different from my four-year-old, who's just so warm and, "I love you, mommy." He doesn't do that. And you know, it's always somebody's else's fault. It's very hard to have a relationship with some-body else, you know. I'm hoping that's going to change with all the things we're going to do. But you know, what kind of person would be attracted to that?

Parents of children with disabilities or developmental delays wondered if their children would ever be able to partner or have children of their own. Keith, whose eleven-year-old daughter was diagnosed with autism when she was five, commented, "[My wife once said to me], '[Our daughter] is probably not ever gonna get married. . . .' I didn't appreciate that very much, but it's prob-ably true. . . . I have to recognize she probably can't . . . and it's kind of painful to think about . . . it's hard emotionally to accept it." Once expressly economic and political, marriage is now thought to be a matter of love and personal ful-fillment.[2] Increasingly, though, marriage is an unrealistic prospect for men and women in low-income communities who never achieve the economic stability deemed necessary for this loftier commitment.[3] Insofar as marriage has become yet another mark of affluence in our highly stratified society, it operated much like a college education in the web of parents' expectations.

It is worth nothing that not all of the parents I interviewed harbored this well-patterned set of assumptions. Adoptive parents were often poised for poten-tial problems at the outset. For example, Carl and Jen have a thirteen-year-old adopted daughter who was diagnosed with an attachment disorder when she was a toddler, and their eight-year-old adopted daughter was diagnosed as hav-ing fetal alcohol effects. These parents expected that their daughters would have problems. Also, the death of their first son had taught them that anything could happen.

> There's like a *billion* things that could go wrong. . . . And I mean, after bursting the
> bubble with the whole pregnancy thing . . . my whole idea of being pregnant was
> this is the step you go through. You get pregnant, you have a baby, blah blah blah.
> And then when this all happened, it was like, whoa! Nobody told me this was
> going to be a problem. So I think that kind of burst our . . . whole "everything goes
> according to plan" [bubble]. You know?

But even though parents like Jen and Carl expected problems, they could not anticipate the full ramifications of their second daughter's fetal alcohol syn-drome. The eight-year-old girl had memory lapses and would forget everything from letters in the alphabet to where she was supposed to wait for her parents to pick her up from school. Every day seemed to present new challenges, so while other parents had to re-examine the benchmarks of an "ordinary" childhood, Jen and Carl found it difficult to harbor any expectations at all. I asked the couple if they ever had regretted the adoption:

JEN: Millions of times.

CARL: Yeah, hindsight is . . . I mean, I wonder, you know, what our family would be like. It would definitely be less chaotic. There's a lot of noise and a lot of trouble because of her behaviors. I don't tend to see a lot of positives. And yeah, we have gone through that. We've admitted it to each other. And that's very true.

JEN: It's not something I'd ever really tell anyone. It's also something we feel like, never in a million years could we reverse that adoption. And I have, out of pure frustration (laughs), looked up what the process is (laughs).

We tend to think of expectations as private or psychological, but in fact they are constitutive elements of social order. Although expectations are the property of individual minds, they bridge subjective and objective social realities and make possible the coordination of human conduct. As foundations for interaction, expectations also provide the groundwork for identity; if we don't know what to expect, it becomes difficult to "locate" ourselves in social space. As Harold Garfinkel demonstrated in his breaching demonstrations, the expectations that keep everyday interactions intact are so deeply taken-for-granted that, like the essence of "normalcy" itself, we recognize them only when they are violated.[4] Thus, the disruption of parents' most basic assumptions about their children's lives temporarily stripped them of the blueprints they had been using for parenthood and family life.

GRIEF

Sociological analyses of grief hinge on the social nature of self; because our selves emerge from and are sustained by our interactions with other people, the disruption of interaction has the potential to damage our internal conversations and images of self in relation to others.[5] Grief is quite literally painful because it is a response to existential harm; the loss of shared meanings that comprise parts of the self is akin to the body's loss of flesh. Mothers' and fathers' anguish was usually just below the surface, permeating their discussion of other topics. Nearly everyone I interviewed expressed intense sorrow. Lauren's twin, ten-year-old adopted daughters have pervasive developmental delays. She sobbed as she said, "I remember an instance . . . [I was] trying to communicate with my husband about how I felt . . . I was in the kitchen and I was explaining something about the girls and their schooling and their problems, and I couldn't talk anymore and so I wrote him a letter . . . and I said, 'I'm dying inside.'" Like Tim, the father I introduced at the beginning of this chapter, many parents used the word "devastating" to describe the emotional impact of their children's difficulties. Deborah, whose twenty-six-year-old son has been an alcoholic since he was fifteen, said,

[There is] real sadness. I mean, just incredible sadness, you know? This is your baby! You brought this little bundle home from the hospital, and it's like the last thing you ever want is for something like that to happen to them. You know the world is not going to be perfect, but you know, you sure as hell don't envision that when you walk out that hospital door. It's devastating (begins to cry). It's absolutely devastating.

As a sociologist, and as someone who did not have children at the time, I had the luxury of asking parents a question that many of them found naïve: why are children's problems so painful? Several parents responded enigmatically, suggesting that I would understand if I had children someday. Others struggled for words. Jessica, whose six-year-old son has trouble controlling his emotions and is aggressive with other children (problems that first manifested when he was four years old), said,

It's such a hard emotion to describe, that connection, that feeling of what you feel for your children. It is overwhelming. I don't know if I can [describe it]! (Laughs) I mean, you'd do anything. You would. You'd do *anything* for them to just make it in this world. And then you see them struggling. It is the saddest thing. It breaks your heart.

Deborah responded in similar terms. When I asked her why her son's alcoholism was so difficult to witness, she said, "I think there's a connection there that will never be broken. Once you're a mother you're always a mother . . . you have these memories of holding this little baby and all these things growing up, there's all this history. Just this rich and very intense history."

Jessica and Deborah's comments highlight the ostensibly sacred quality of the parent–child relationship. People often describe the experience of parenthood in spiritual or religious terms,[6] and, in the contemporary Western world, the parent–child bond is thought to be one of the strongest and most permanent bonds that a person can experience. Some of the women I interviewed indicated that this connection was specifically maternal. "Once a mother, always a mother," Deborah asserted. While it is true that the emotional culture of intensive mothering essentializes the deep affective connection between mother and child,[7] most of the fathers I interviewed also said they felt a strong emotional bond with their children. Keith's eleven-year-old daughter was diagnosed with autism when she was five. When I asked him if anything about fatherhood had surprised him, he responded that,

[Before you have children] you don't appreciate the extent to which you'll do anything for *your kids*. . . . And then you don't understand how difficult it's going to be when your kid is having problems. . . . [You think] "We have to do every-thing we can! What can I do today?" You know, it's this kind of consuming thing. "This is someone I have to take care of. I want to take care of. I need to do what-ever I can for this person." You don't quite appreciate that, I think, until you have your own kids. . . . You would throw yourself in front of a bus [for your children].

Seth made similar comments. His fourteen-year-old daughter had been addicted to drugs and had run away multiple times, though she is now nineteen years old, sober, and living at home. When Seth and his wife made the decision to send their daughter to an out-of-state therapeutic boarding school, he had to physi-cally force her into the car and drive her, against her will, to the school site. He said it was the hardest day of his life.

I would rather have lost a limb, you know? I don't know why. When they're born, they weasel their way so deeply into your heart, they're a part of you. Physically, they're just so much *who you are*, and you care . . . you do so many things, you make so many accommodations in your life to take care of that. . . . If you're a parent who really cares about your kids—and most people are—it's not a ques-tion . . . nothing else matters. I mean, literally. Burn my house down. Everything in it. I don't care. Give me my kids. . . . And most parents I think feel that way about their kids.

During interviews, parents repeatedly described their children as parts of them-selves. When I asked Andrea why her daughter's drug and alcohol problems had been so painful, she replied, "It's like having a part of you . . . this person that was a part of you, turn out in this totally unpredicted way." As an extension of this conceptualization, mothers and fathers said that their relationships with their children were characterized by a deep empathy. They experienced pain whenever their children experienced pain. Steve and Marie, who discovered six months prior to our interview that their seventeen-year-old daughter is a cocaine addict, both cried openly during their three-hour interview. When I asked why the discovery of their daughter's addiction had been so painful, they replied,

STEVE: I think as a parent you hurt when your kids hurt . . . and there's no way for me to give you an appreciation for the mindset, the pressure that was weighing on [our daughter's] head. . . . It was incredible. No seventeen-year-old kid should *ever* have to go through that.
MARIE: It's sharing her pain.

Parents also said that watching their children reminded them of their own childhood, an identification that generated strong emotions. For example, Jason, whose son was diagnosed with autism when he was eighteen months old, said that it was gut-wrenching to think that other children might tease his six-year-old autistic son. He explained,

> I think part of it is we were all kids, and we all had our situations in school where . . . school wasn't so great, socially. I remember a couple situations where older kids just sort of singled me out in a class . . . and I still remember those painful experiences. So I think part of my gut-wrench is just from my own personal experience of, "Oh, god, I know what that feels like. I remember what that feels like." And you know, you don't want that for your kids.

The gut-wrenching quality of parents' grief reflects the social nature of self and the lived experience of loss as sociologists conceive of it. In this case, the profound degree to which parents' selves were joined to the selves of their children led parents to experience a physical, visceral sorrow.

Unlike other participants, the parents whose teenaged children had drug or alcohol problems (or who were otherwise rebellious) suffered through the additional pain of estrangement. Such parents viewed their grief as markedly different from that of parents whose children had disabilities, as I learned when I attended an Al-Anon meeting for parents whose children are alcoholics or drug addicts. When I explained to the group that I was interviewing parents whose children have a wide range of problems, one mother exclaimed that having a developmentally disabled child would be preferable to having one who is an addict. I was puzzled by her comment and did not have the opportunity to ask her what she meant. But when I interviewed Matt and Sarah, they echoed this mother's sentiment. Matt's seventeen-year-old biological son has had drug and alcohol problems since he was fifteen. Sarah's thirteen-year-old biological son was diagnosed with cerebral palsy at birth and is severely disabled. The couple, who has been married for ten years, explained,

MATT: As complex and painful and difficult [our situation with our son with disabilities] is, we have, more emotional issues with [our other son]. With [our son with disabilities], you can kind of package [him] up, stick him in his room, put some music on, and breathe. He's not coming in your face going, "You're an asshole because you won't let me drive my car" . . . the child with disabilities loves you.
SARAH: He doesn't reject us.
MATT: He doesn't reject us.
SARAH: Rejection is really . . . horrible.

Matt and Sarah's comments highlight a distinctive aspect of the losses suffered by the parents of teenaged children whose "problems" were not understood in terms of disease or disability. Such parents viewed their children as partly responsible for their own behavior, and this attribution of "intentionality," though it reduced parents' own ostensible culpability, was especially painful. Unlike parents whose children's problems became apparent early in life, the parents of teenaged children had established relatively mature relationships with their sons and daughters. The notion that their children were willingly disobeying or rejecting them caused additional sorrow.

Pervasive uncertainty complicated parents' losses because it prevented them from realigning their expectations. In some cases, children's problems did not automatically preclude particular futures, and parents had no idea what to expect. When I interviewed Steve and Marie, their daughter was at a therapeutic boarding school. She was scheduled to return home that same month, and it was not clear whether or not she would continue to have problems or would be able to begin college in the fall as she had planned. Steve said,

> [Our daughter is] coming back in two weeks, and I don't know what she's gonna do on the second day she's back. . . . We cannot be with her twenty-four hours a day, seven days a week going forward . . . [and] here's a kid that's supposed to go off to college next September. . . . We don't know if that's gonna happen. . . . That's gonna be the next bridge to cross.

Parents were sometimes unsure whether or not it was more appropriate to hope or grieve. As I mentioned in an earlier chapter, Claire's nine-year-old son was diagnosed with autism when he was three, and she put him in an intensive, in-home treatment program when he was diagnosed. She had held onto the hope that early intervention would essentially "normalize" him, and she described it as "heartbreaking" when she realized he would remain autistic. She started to cry as she explained how hope had prolonged her grief.

> Some kids really do come through it. So you decide your kid is gonna be one of those. So you fight like hell, and then you have what they call the second heartbreak, which is what happened with [my son], definitely. Because after you get through with the program, you see he's not gonna be saved.

Parents like Steve and Claire experienced what psychologists sometimes call an "ambiguous loss," or a loss that occurs when someone is "there, but not there."[8] Originally used to describe emotionally distant fathers in the 1970s, the concept has been extended to describe losses that defy closure, such as when a family member is missing but presumed dead. Here, Pauline Boss explains how ambiguous loss presents unique challenges for the bereaved.

Ambiguous loss is the most stressful loss because it defies resolution. . . . With a clear-cut loss, there is more clarity—a death certificate, mourning rituals, and the opportunity to honor and dispose remains. With ambiguous loss, none of these markers exists. . . . Decisions are put on hold, daily tasks are undone. . . . The irresolvable situation tends to block cognition, block coping and stress management, and freeze the grief process.[9]

As Boss suggests, uncertainty prolonged parents' grief, sometimes indefinitely, and made this aspect of their troubles particularly difficult to overcome.

Grief compounded parents' troubles in two ways. First, parents' pain was so great that it seemed to them, at times, to be unbearable. Women's advocacy care on children's behalf was, in part, motivated by a desire to escape their sorrow. Not only did this contribute to the disruption of routines and resulting exhaustion that I described earlier, but, as some mothers said in retrospect, it sustained false hopes and made their sadness more difficult to manage. Lisa's nine-year-old son and five-year-old daughter were both born with hyperinsulinism. Her son sustained severe brain damage from the condition shortly after birth. Lisa said that it was not until she stopped trying to "fix" her son that she was able to cope with her grief. She stated,

I think [I spent] so many years . . . trying to fix him, thinking, "How can we help this. . . ." I mean, I looked into *everything*. You know, homeopathic medication, hyperbaric oxygen therapy, I went to Stanford, I went to UCSF, and I think back then I was spending so much time trying to fix him and trying to make him better that at some point, I feel like you get to a point where you go, "This is him. Let's just work with who he is," and get rid of that energy trying to go here and there. . . . So yes, it always hurts. Yes, it's always there. But I think back then it was harder because I was doing so much, and I felt the pressure around me to do things. And now that I've gotten to this point . . . I'm just more, "Let's take what we have right now and move on."

The second way that grief served to amplify parents' troubles was through further stigmatization. It is normative for people in late-modern, Western societies to offer sympathy to those in trouble, but tolerance for others' misery is finite.[10] As their sorrow stretched on, some parents felt as though they had exhausted the sympathy reserves of family members and friends. Lauren, for example, received the explicit message that she was talking too much about her children's problems. Her twin, ten-year-old adopted daughters have pervasive developmental delays, and she first became concerned about their development when they were three. Lauren said,

I have worn out relatives, specifically my mother and my sister. . . . Sometimes they're as blatant as, "I don't want to talk about it anymore." So then I'll say, "Fine, if you don't let me vent in any way I can, and as much as I can, I'm just not gonna tell you anything." And that's when I say I feel kind of alone.

As this quote demonstrates, parents' grief sometimes became its own source of stigma and isolation. Their sorrow, it seemed, gave way to greater trouble.

SELF-DOUBT, GUILT, AND ANXIETY

Intensive mothering is not simply a set of ideas about what mothers should *do*; it is also a set of beliefs about how mothers should *feel*.[11] Guilt and anxiety, it seems, are part and parcel of this emotional culture.[12] Both the men and women I interviewed experienced these emotions intensely; children's problems directly challenged their childrearing capabilities. Across children's ages and problem type, most parents described pervasive self-doubt as an inevitable, taken-for-granted part of their circumstances.

Many wondered whether or not they had caused their children's problems. When I asked Andrea, for example, if she blamed herself for her nineteen-year-old daughter's excessive use of drugs and alcohol, she said, "I think you always wonder. 'What did I do or didn't I do that may have caused this? Did I miss something?' You always do." Matt, whose seventeen-year-old biological son has had drug and alcohol problems since he was fifteen, made similar comments. He stated,

I don't want to say it's my fault because it's not my fault . . . [but] I think you always go, "What can I do different?" or "What could I have done? At this moment in time, what could I have done differently?" And so, you never know. . . . "What did I do wrong then to make him this way now?"
. . . I don't know. You just don't know.

Some parents were plagued with quite specific concerns about what they might have done wrong. When children had congenital disabilities, mothers questioned their prenatal care and whether or not they caused damage to their children in utero. Kathy, whose six-year-old son was diagnosed with cerebral palsy before his first birthday, commented,

For a long time I blamed myself. . . . I was like, "What did I do?" I was searching within my nine months of pregnancy and thinking, "Okay, what did I do wrong? Maybe when I did this," or, "Maybe I didn't drink enough water," or "Maybe I didn't exercise."

Daniel thought that he might have caused his son's problems by fighting too much with his ex-spouse while she was pregnant. Now eighteen years old, Daniel's son began exhibiting intellectual and social delays when he was four and has been diagnosed with auditory processing disorder and attention deficit/hyperactivity disorder. When I asked Daniel if he had ever felt guilty about his son's ongoing learning problems, he said,

> Yeah! Oh, absolutely . . . and I've thought about this from the womb. We never fought physically by any stretch. But we fought verbally all the time. Especially toward the end . . . the fighting was incredibly intense when [he] was in the womb. And I've thought, how did that affect him? I believe that—that it can and could. . . . I felt guilty about that.

Instead of automatically releasing parents from culpability, biological accounts of children's problems sometimes led to further self-doubt or guilt.[13] Some parents felt guilty about having passed along "bad genes," for example. Joan's fifteen-year-old son began showing symptoms of mental illness when he was eleven. Doctors think he may develop schizophrenia. Joan believes that her son inherited a predisposition for mental illness from her side of the family, something that she used to feel bad about. She explained,

> I felt that it was my fault. And the reason I thought it was my fault is because of my genetic background. This seems to be something that does affect the males in our family from the same father. The girls are fine, we're the strong [ones]. . . . So I blamed myself for a long time.

Even adoptive parents experienced self-doubt about children's ostensibly biomedical problems. Jen, whose second adopted daughter was diagnosed with fetal alcohol syndrome, found it more difficult to bond with her than with her other three children. This made her feel incredibly guilty. When one of the girl's schoolteachers noticed a behavioral change, she asked Jen if anything was "going on at home." Jen recalled, "*That* really threw me, actually for days. Because then I thought, 'It's all because it's been different with her!' . . . it was horrible. It scared me. Because I thought, 'Oh gosh, I'm not doing something right,' you know? Yeah, I totally blamed myself. Oh, I was a mess."

Some parents firmly believed that bad parenting practices contributed to their children's problems, though this was not common. For example Joel, whose thirteen-year-old daughter attempted suicide when she was eleven, believed that his daughter's ongoing problems in school were partly the result of his and his wife's inconsistent rule setting. He said,

I do feel a little bit guilty that we've been such poor models for [our children] on how to have a non-dysfunctional marriage and household. . . . We've screwed up royally, you know, in a lot of respects. Our limits have never been consistently enforced, and that's a big mistake. And I know that doesn't occur in every household. There are households where parents are able to be consistent. But not ours.

For some parents whose children had drug and alcohol problems, guilt stemmed not from a perceived failure to discipline, but from a perceived over-involvement or over-investment in their children's lives. Mary and Phil's seventeen-year-old son began using and selling drugs three years ago. He was diagnosed with ADHD when he was in the sixth-grade and has also been in trouble for fighting. Phil wondered if his son had gotten into trouble because he had placed too much pressure on him to achieve in sports. He stated, "Oh, it's been a year and a half, two years of guilt. . . . I'm a huge sports fan. And I had a kid who was a pretty good athlete. And I've often asked myself, 'Did I push him too much? Did he think that was the only thing that was important to me about him?' And I haven't gotten that impression from him through all of this. But there is constant guilt." Phil's wife, Mary, felt guilty about their son's problems for similar reasons. She said,

I totally felt guilty. I was sure it was everything I had done wrong, though I didn't know what it was. If we had it to do over again, I know a lot of things I'd do different . . . [our son] was never abused or neglected or anything. My kids have always come first. Maybe *too* much. . . . I just think that I've overindulged them.

Parents also worried about how they were responding to their children's troubles and whether or not they were doing everything they could to alleviate them. Just like grief, guilt and the fear of future guilt animated women's advocacy care and, in turn, contributed to the disruption of parents' routines. Claire, whose nine-year-old son was diagnosed with autism when he was three, accounted for her efforts in the following way:

[You have to fight] to get the *best* services possible because better services usually mean better outcome. And what I hear from parents who didn't put up the fight . . . is they live with guilt. *Terrible* guilt. Because they think, "What if I had? What if I'd gotten [a home program]? What if I'd gotten those thirty hours per week as opposed to ten hours in the state preschool?" Because if you miss the window of opportunity, you'll never know.

Phil made a similar comment about the choice to send his son, Adam, to a therapeutic boarding school. Adam had been using drugs and getting in trouble for a few years, and his parents had tried a number of treatment options, including private counseling and an outpatient recovery program. Their son's bad behavior had continued, and Phil and Mary were at their wits' end when they decided to send him to an out-of-state wilderness program and boarding school designed to treat teens with substance abuse problems. Adam tried to run away when he learned of his parents' intentions, and they had to forcibly restrain him when representatives from the school arrived to transport him to the wilderness site. Phil said that part of the decision to proceed was driven by his and his wife's desire to avoid future guilt. He commented,

> Part of the thing about sending him to [the boarding school], sending him to the wilderness, was that if we didn't do that, if things didn't turn out okay, we would have the constant feeling that we should have done that. Despite all the hardship it caused and how difficult it was to go through [that] . . . [if we had] let him leave, we would have had to live with it. Now, if something happens when he comes back, we're gonna continue to make efforts, but we will know we tried awfully hard. And part of that is the guilt you would feel.

Ever-present self-doubt seemed to stem, in part, from the notion that parents were solely responsible for children and their problems. Many of the mothers and fathers I interviewed expressed disillusionment with public institutions and rejected the notion that they could trust experts to do what was in their children's best interests. Bill, whose sixteen-year-old son developed a seizure disorder when he was five months old and now has developmental disabilities, explained,

> We got a lot of bad information from the doctors. . . . We're just parents, you know, we don't know. And that's unfortunate because you put the doctors on such a pedestal. And now we don't, now we kick 'em off the pedestal. And you know, we know doctors are jerks and stuff. We know that now, after going through this journey.

Even those who trusted their children's doctors and teachers believed that when it came to treating children's problems, parents had to do the legwork. There was a pervasive sense that in the absence of intensive caregiving, children would be utterly lost. Olivia and Jerry's ten-year-old adopted son has a congenital brain injury that has caused him myriad learning and behavioral problems. These parents had the following exchange:

OLIVIA: The stuff is out there that you need, but you have to go and get it. Nobody is gonna bring it to you.

JERRY: You have to go find it, yep . . .

OLIVIA: You just have to do it. Because you know what? . . . half those people that are in jail now have ADD (laughs). . . . You know, fifty percent, ADD, and nobody helped them. Because they didn't recognize it for whatever reason. So ask questions, ask questions, ask questions. That's what you've gotta do.

This heavy sense of personal responsibility is characteristic of the risk culture I described in Chapter 2. Public discourse about how to best manage risk is suffused with neoliberalism. "Scientists, doctors, and government institutions emphasize individual responsibility," Joan Wolf explains, "and good citizens are idealized as those who take care of themselves and exercise personal control."[14] This is particularly true in the United States, where anxiety about childrearing is bolstered by a lack of formal and informal support. When it comes to family matters, many industrialized countries have rejected the individualism that still characterizes policy in the U.S.[15] Thus, parents' sense of having to "go it alone" no doubt contributed to their self-doubt and guilt.

Given this enormous burden of parental responsibility, guilt and the fear of future guilt compelled action. But how much was enough? And which treatments were the "correct" treatments? Questions like these fed parents' anxieties, and their self-doubt was a partner to constant worrying. Lauren first became concerned about her twin, ten-year-old adopted daughters' developmental delays when they were three. When I asked her whether or not she felt guilty about her daughters' conditions, she began by questioning things she had done in the past. Her narrative moved seamlessly from past doubts to current anxieties.

Maybe I should have read more to [the twins]. Maybe we should have gone on nature hikes everyday. . . . I always say, "Did I do enough?" Maybe we need to make another batch of cookies and they'll learn. Or instead of hauling them to therapy five days of week, we'll just do it [once a week] . . . and then [I think], I need to go out and find some other test or some other assessment for them to do. Maybe I'm just not doing enough to identify what it is that will help them learn.

Having disrupted whatever confidence parents might have previously had, children's problems generated a flood of seemingly unanswerable questions about what parents had done, what they should be doing, what was happening now, and what would happen in the future. When parents believed that their children could not fend for themselves, these anxieties persisted long after they had stopped looking for treatments. Tim explained,

Well the number one thing I worry about is, what's gonna happen to [our son] when [my spouse] and I aren't here anymore? Because even if we create—and we will—some type of fall-back position, some place where he could live, you know, funded, a living-trust, whatever. . . . That's still not going to replace the vital role, the emotional role, that [my spouse] and I play in [his] life. We're his world . . . and so that worries me.

GENDER, COMMITMENT, AND EMOTION

The literature on intensive parenting and previous studies on raising children with disabilities focus almost exclusively on women's experiences, paying close attention to the simultaneously regressive and progressive elements of late-modern, middle-class maternal practices.[16] Without a doubt, some aspects of parents' experiences are highly gendered and place women at a disadvantage; mothers perceived stigma more often than fathers did, invested themselves fully in the work of "problem" identification and problem treatment, and played a pivotal role in the construction of trouble. However, the dearth of men's first-hand accounts in previous literature might lead us to believe that fathers are altogether absent, emotionally, if not physically, from children and childrearing.

The data I have presented thus far in this chapter demonstrate how misleading this is. Masculine privilege did not spare men from the emotional fallout stemming from children's problems. Men, as a group, may have spent less time dwelling on difficult feelings during their interviews, but fathers like Tim, Steve, and Seth openly discussed how devastated they were. Several men wept during our conversations. For the most part, when I observed differences between mothers' and fathers' emotional experiences, those differences were a matter of degree, not of kind. When asked directly, some married couples emphasized emotional similarity rather than gender difference, stating that they were equally troubled by children's problems but expressed and managed their emotions differently. Mary and Phil's seventeen-year-old son was diagnosed with ADHD when he was in the sixth-grade, began using and selling drugs three years ago, and has also been in trouble for fighting. Mary said that leading up to their son's departure for a therapeutic boarding school, she could not eat or sleep and had lost twenty-five pounds. However, when I asked her and Phil if one of them had suffered more than the other, I was surprised when they said no. Phil explained,

We deal with things a little differently. I tend to internalize . . . but I've suffered the same things. There's been nights I'd just sit on the couch and wait for him to come home. She would say, "Why don't you come up, you're not doing any good." . . . I still think about things constantly. So I can't put a degree on things.

Nonetheless, consistent with the narratives of denial I discussed in Chapter 2, some women believed that men refused to face the difficult emotions associated with children's problems. Kathy, whose husband declined an interview, said that he had "blocked" his feelings. Their six-year-old son was diagnosed with cerebral palsy before his first birthday. Kathy explained,

> [My husband] didn't understand. He wasn't going through it like I was. He's like, "What's the big deal? That's just [our son]." . . . I think too, he's blocked some of that emotion . . . just being a guy. I've talked to other parents [whose children have disabilities], and they're like, "Yeah, my husband did the same thing" (laughs). You know, "It's just [our son]." My other friend [said], "I got the same thing."

Fathers occasionally made similar comments, drawing on popular stereotypes to characterize men as emotionally simplistic. The needs of Matt and Sarah's developmentally disabled son limit the couple's ability to relax, travel, and spend time alone. After Sarah said that the loss of freedom was still sometimes painful for her, I asked Matt how he felt. The couple had the following exchange:

MATT: I don't go [in a feminine voice], "Oh, I'm feeling pensive." Or, "I'm feeling this," [I don't have] these emotional words that you can kind of go, "I'm feeling this," or "I'm feeling that." It's like . . . what did I say?
SARAH: [You said] you had three emotions . . . angry, tired, or happy (laughs) . . .
MATT: Happy, tired, or pissed off . . . it's like colors for men, right? There's black, there's white, there's red, there's blue, there's green. Mauve? Nobody knows what it is. And so . . . is it mauve? I don't know.

Despite resorting to gender-essentializing discourse when talking about these emotional differences, parents' accounts suggest an explanation that relies on what identity theorists call "commitment." Commitment refers to "the degree to which persons' relationships to others in their networks depend on possessing a particular identity and role."[17] Commitment shapes, and is shaped by, the salience—or relative importance—of a particular identity. The more a person's relationships depend on performing a particular role, in other words, the more salient the identity associated with that role, and vice-versa.[18] In this view, emotions serve as a kind of weathervane; challenges to a salient identity result in negative emotions that, in turn, encourage the person to realign her conduct, reduce her commitment to the role, or redefine the situation.[19]

As previous chapters make clear, most women's daily lives were, relative to fathers', more fully predicated on child rearing. In other words, women's "commitment" to parenthood was greater than that of most fathers'. It follows that the disruption of childrearing patterns—taken-for-granted meanings, routines, relationships—had greater ramifications for women's emotional worlds. Parents' comments lend support to this argument. Keith, for example, said that his wife Valerie shouldered much of the emotional impact of their eleven-year-old daughter's condition. She was diagnosed with autism when she was five. Keith explained,

> [Valerie] was *a mess*. Because she was the one who was on the front line dealing with [the healthcare system].... You know, there would be days where she would have waited on hold with the insurance company for an hour or something and then they can't tell her or they gotta swap it off to the next person or whatever. I mean she was just very upset a lot of the time, having to deal with that.... I think that that made it difficult for her because we were having to deal with the fact that [our daughter] has problems.... I think it was easier for me.... I wasn't completely immersed in that all of the time. I went to work. And even if work was miserable, it wasn't being immersed in that.

Rather than viewing his wife's grief as a natural maternal expression, Keith saw it as a consequence of a gendered division of domestic labor. Performing the role of stay-at-home mother meant that Valerie spent hours each day engaged in advocacy care. Keith, in contrast, could escape into his role performance as a lawyer. In his words, his grief was not as intense because he was not as "immersed" in tasks of child rearing. I had a similar exchange with Peter, whose six-year-old son has trouble controlling his emotions and is aggressive with other children. These problems first manifested when the boy was four years old.

ARA: In terms of just the emotional impacts of this ... do you think it was more or less difficult for one of you than the other, in terms of you and [your spouse]?
PETER: I mean, she was being the primary caregiver. She probably dealt with more frustration than I did. I mean, there were times when I know she had some really difficult days and because I wasn't there, she wasn't able just to kind of hand him off and walk away.

From a sociological perspective, emotions are not just internal experiences that exist independently of circumstance. Indeed, parents frequently said that grief was *evoked* by certain images, circumstances, or interactions. Tim said that he experiences pain whenever he sees "other fathers doing [things] with their sons." Similarly, Sarah said that she lamented the loss of her professional aspirations when she sees "pictures of business women, or ... different women doing different things." It is likely that mothers encountered such emotional "triggers" more often than their spouses because routine caretaking brought them into situations—such as doctor's offices, school settings, or play dates—that called their grief, guilt, self-doubt, and anxiety to the fore.

Previous sociological literature on motherhood relies strongly on the concept of "ideology" when examining the gendered terrain of parenthood in the contemporary United States.[20] In other words, sociologists account for gendered parenting practices and gendered emotions by citing a culturally pervasive set of *ideas* about what good mothers think, feel, and do. The ideology of intensive mothering consists of three beliefs: mothers naturally make the best primary caregivers, good mothers value their children above and beyond all other interests and obligations, and good mothering consists of "child-centered, expert-guided, emotionally absorbing, labor-intensive, and financially expensive" methods.[21] The emotional dimensions of this ideology include unconditional love, confidence, protectiveness, moral conviction, and attachment.[22]

Clearly, ideas or beliefs about what mothers and fathers should feel are at work in parents' experiences and expressions of grief, guilt, and anxiety. The very notion that women are more emotionally complex than men is an ideological matter, and such assumptions frame how men and women make sense of their emotions. However, my data suggest that the day-to-day practices of childrearing—and the interactions in which those practices are embedded— also play a key role. In many cases, it is not ideas or beliefs but the *doing of parenthood* that generates the difficult emotions stemming from children's problems. These emotions look gender-specific because women spend more time performing childcare. In this way, parents' emotions serve to maintain the ideology of intensive mothering and its associated emotional culture.

Ultimately, women's greater immersion in the day-to-day tasks of childrearing (and the emotions that those routines and interactions cultivated) generated a gendered division of emotional labor where some mothers aimed to "help" fathers experience and express emotion in ways deemed appropriate by the emotional culture of good mothering. Like Kathy, Joan believed that her husband, Sergio, had not yet been able to face the fact that their fifteen-year-old son suffered from a mental illness. "My husband is a little less open," she said, "and I think a little less connected to his own . . . emotions and feelings . . . I think he was raised in a way that . . . boys don't cry, and you be a tough man . . . and he's a good person, I just think to this day he still is kind of frozen with, 'What do I do?'" At first Joan tried to instruct Sergio, encouraging him to spend more time with their son and be more emotionally forthcoming. When that did not work, she arranged for him to see a therapist. She explained,

> I think my husband is in a depression right now. And I think, um, it's . . . you
> know, the first layer is anger and resentment, and underneath that is sadness and

loss. And underneath that is a little boy who didn't have the father that he needed and wanted. And I think until he deals with that . . . he is going to continue to be resentful and impatient and he's doing a disservice to his son and to himself. I know he loves [our son], I just don't think he's aware of how he needs to help [him]. . . . And when the suggestions come from me, you know, I'm his wife, and he gets resentful. So if it comes from another man in therapy, I think it would be better. I'm hoping that in the long run that [therapy] will really help.

When I interviewed Sergio five months later and asked what advice he would give to other fathers in his situation, it was clear he was doing his best to adopt a therapeutic narrative: "[You have to] open your eyes, your heart, your mind. And get some therapy. Not saying that they need it, but just open their minds up more so that they can see what's going on. Because if you don't and try to do it yourself, you'll be doing more damage than good. Um, therapy has been very very good for me."

As I discuss in the next chapter, women like Joan were exposed to narratives about "healthy grieving" in support and advocacy groups, as well as in the course of personal therapy. These narratives led them to believe that men's handling of emotion was pathological. In turn, women often tried to act as their spouse's emotional mentors. Bill—who had at different times been the primary caretaker for his developmentally disabled son—said that his wife had encouraged him to grieve. He recalled,

I didn't understand the grief cycle for a long time. My wife had some counseling help. And of course, being the man, "I don't want counseling help. I don't need no counseling," and stuff. And she kept saying, "You've gotta grieve. You've gotta grieve." I said, "Grieve? He's not dead." Because I only equated the grief cycle with death. And it wasn't until I heard it three and four and five times that I finally said, "Oh, I understand it now. Yeah, okay."

In addition to washing dishes, doing the laundry, and other concrete chores, family members perform "emotion work" for one another. Emotion work occurs when people attempt to align their emotional experiences or expressions with culturally appropriate ways of feeling.[23] People perform emotion work on themselves, but they also can work upon the "untoward" emotions of others.[24] The demonstration of affection, encouragement, appreciation, and empathy is a central part of the carework that family members are expected to perform for one another.[25] From this perspective, women's emotion work on behalf of fathers is yet another manifestation of an unequal division of household labor.

Just as children's problems undermined the micro-social structure of daily life by disrupting parents' routines and relationships, they troubled parents' expectations and engendered a painful mix of grief, guilt, and anxiety. As illustrated here, the emotional features of parents' experiences were not mere responses to trouble but contributed to its manifestation by further alienating parents from family members and friends and by encouraging mothers, in particular, to find suitable remedies at any cost. Many parents said that their children's problems had resulted in a period of "depression." Although some used this term casually, referring to a period of deep sadness rather than a clinical diagnosis per se, twenty of the parents in this study did seek help from psychologists, psychiatrists, or family therapists when trying to cope and come to terms with children's problems. In a culture that strongly pathologizes negative emotion and tends to reduce all human experience to one's own psychology, the language of "depression" was, perhaps, the only one parents had for trying to understand what they were going through. As I argue in the next chapter, however, parents' experiences are best understood using a sociological framework, and their emotional turmoil can be more accurately described as an expression, not of depression, but of anomie.

6 • DISRUPTED SELVES, MAKING SENSE, AND MAKING DO

Andrea, a registered nurse in her late fifties, volunteered for an interview after hearing about my research at an Al-Anon meeting. Al-Anon is an offshoot of Alcoholics Anonymous designed to support the family members and close friends of alcoholics, and the meeting I attended was comprised mostly of parents troubled by their teenaged children's misconduct. Andrea's daughter Lily was nineteen at the time and had spent the better part of two years in out-of-state, therapeutic boarding schools. There were times when Andrea thought that the programs were working and that her daughter was overcoming the defiance, aggression, and substance abuse that had caused terrible upheaval at home. However, after a series of rule violations and an incidence of drug use, Lily was expelled before she could graduate. When her daughter returned home, Andrea asked her to live elsewhere; by then Lily had turned eighteen, and her parents had decided to limit her financial support. When I talked with Andrea over tea at her dining room table, she explained that Lily was now unemployed, living with a boyfriend, and recently had been arrested under charges of domestic violence.

Andrea was absolutely bewildered by her daughter's behavior. She herself had grown up in less than privileged circumstances. A Chinese-American child from a family of seven, she thought that her parents had done "a horrible job." Nonetheless, she and her siblings had "turned out really well, successful." In contrast, Lily was an only child. Andrea was an attentive mother and had been involved in Lily's grade school activities. She and her husband had been "very caring and loving" and had even moved to a different community so that Lily could attend a well-funded public school. Part of what was so troubling about her daughter's delinquency was its unfamiliarity. Andrea marveled at her daughter's departure from what she considered to be the norm.

Going to college. Finding a career. Not getting into trouble. I mean, [Lily's choices are] so foreign to me. Having a really productive life . . . to me that's being happy, you know? Being able to feel accomplishment and achievement. And feeling proud of what you've been able to do. Doing well. I mean, somehow her motivations were not at all in line with mine, what I grew up with.

The most difficult years had been before Andrea and her husband decided to send their daughter away for treatment. In Andrea's words, Lily had become "hardened" and uncommunicative. She often disappeared, staying out until the wee hours of the morning and leaving Andrea to imagine where she was and what she was doing. "I couldn't stop worrying about her and what was gonna happen to her," Andrea remembered. "This was a period where it's full of nightmares." After Andrea outlined the history of Lily's problems, I asked her to speak about what those early years had been like for her, socially and emotionally. She underscored her profound sense of being cut off from other people.

I was, like, near tears the entire time. . . . [from] the embarrassment, the shame, isolation. Not having anybody that you could really talk to or share any of these problems with. . . . The community made it very easy for me because they basically ignored me. I didn't have a single phone call from any other parent. When [Lily] didn't show up for volleyball the following year, not one parent called me to say, "I understand you might be having some difficulties, is there anything I can do?" Or, "Anytime you want to talk." Not one . . . it was only when I started to reach out to certain parents that the word got out . . . but I could not do it while I was having all the turmoil and the pain . . . I just couldn't. I didn't know what to say.

When Lily left for treatment, Andrea and her husband sought counseling to work through marital problems that had been compounded by their daughter's delinquency. Andrea also started to attend Al-Anon meetings, where she met parents in similar situations. Employing the framework of "codependency," Al-Anon encouraged Andrea to gain distance from her daughter's problems. Over time, she learned how to accept her situation.

I could easily go back to that place . . . [but] I've learned to manage my fears better. And my husband and I have been able to repair and help sustain our relationship. . . . I did go to the Al-Anon meetings, and you learn that there's some times that you do have to detach. . . . I do worry still, a little bit. I try not to . . . I try to sort of distance myself and say, "Okay." I have to remind myself, "It's her life. It's not my life." But there's still that part that hurts and hopes.

Andrea unequivocally said that coping with Lily's problems has been the most difficult thing that she has ever had to do. At the same time, she feels as though the last several years have made her a better person. She explained,

> I'm grateful for the fact that I feel that I've grown a lot . . . and I think I'm a more sensitive person. I'm a more compassionate person. I try to live more presently. I used to be really really bad about living in the future. And planning things out. A lot. And there's nothing like this kind of a lesson that lets you know that you just can't plan some things in life. . . . I think this is her path, it's my path. And we're both learning to live with it. And learning, learning, learning to live. And learning to love. And [with a deep intake of breath] learning about life.

These comments demonstrate how, beyond losing the child she imagined she would have, Andrea had to let go of an overarching narrative that placed productivity and accomplishment at the center of a happy life. She had played by the rules. She had worked hard to garner an education, find a meaningful vocation, and provide her daughter with a loving home. In this particular story, cherished by so many middle-class Americans, Lily would follow her mother's upward trajectory and emerge from childhood a "successful" and "happy" middle-class woman. But Lily's actual trajectory, delineated by unemployment, substance abuse, violence, and legal trouble, renders that story implausible. Andrea has learned to tell a new story about herself, a person who has become more sensitive and compassionate. She is no longer the "planner" she used to be but instead finds wisdom in living in the moment.

In this chapter, I examine how parents' troubles culminated in self-disruption and led them to re-examine what it means to live a "good life." Like Andrea, the mothers and fathers in this book could no longer sustain the narratives they had woven about themselves and their families. The expectations, routines, and relationships that had sustained those stories were no longer strong enough to support them. This generated within parents a sense of otherness. As I explain in this chapter, parents' troubles associated them with underprivileged families, and this diminished their sense of belonging to an imagined community of "normal," middle-class Americans. Moreover, the experience of deep hardship—in Andrea's words, the realization that "you just can't plan some things in life"— shook some parents to the core. Men and women whose children had severe and intractable problems sometimes faced an existential crisis that led them to question or radically alter their worldviews.

It is true that parents suffered tremendously. Family trouble manifested in their minds and bodies, and many exhibited "depression" and "anxiety." However, I argue here that the sociological term "anomie" more aptly captures their experiences. Parents' inner turmoil, I contend, was seeded not in their individual psyches but stemmed, instead, from fractures in their connection to social life. In the language of "family trouble," children's problems had upended the patterns of social life that had provided these middle-class parents with a basic sense of security and well-being.

Not all parents emerged with coherent narratives that bridged old expectations with the new. At the time of these interviews, at least, some participants were simply trying to get by from day-to-day, aware that they were no longer who they used to be but unsure about the people they were becoming. But others, like Andrea, talked about themselves as having come through to the other side of despair and hopelessness. Children's problems sometimes afforded participants new and unexpected opportunities to see themselves as "good parents." In a few cases, whether due to treatment or the mere passing of time, children's conditions and behaviors improved, and parents' troubles diminished. More frequently, however, children's problems persisted and support groups helped parents to craft new stories that re-anchored them to social life. Like Andrea, parents who participated in Al-Anon learned to distance themselves from what they came to view as their children's "bad choices." In support groups for parents with special needs, parents came to view their children as different, rather than disappointing. By forming relationships with other parents whose children had problems, parents eased their feelings of isolation. They also developed a sense of gratitude for having suffered. In fact, many parents echoed Andrea's comments, saying that although the hardships associated with children's problems were more painful than anything they had experienced before, they were better people for having lived through them. Thus, parents' troubles were a matter of biographical revision, as well as biographical disruption.

BIOGRAPHICAL DISRUPTION AND REVISION

Although we are our own storytellers, the tales we spin about ourselves do not emerge simply from our own imaginations. Our biographical narratives are tethered to everyday events, and they require the people around us to play along.[1] Parents and children are role partners, which means that children's performances set the parameters for the stories that parents could tell about themselves as mothers or fathers. Because children were such pivotal characters in parents' biographies, they also had the power to shift parents' identities well beyond parenthood itself.

Several mothers said that, before they had children, they imagined that they would be excellent parents. However, the stigma of "bad parenting" made it difficult for them to perform and to view themselves as "good mothers." Andrea laughed as she explained, "Here you're trying to be the perfect parent, to do as well as you can. And no matter what you do, it's not turning out that way. I mean, I tried to be perfect. But you know, that doesn't mean anybody else is gonna want to be!" As this quote highlights, being a "perfect" mother was contingent, for some women, upon having a "perfect" child. The loss of such a child disrupted the narrative that "good" mothering yields "good" children. Women whose children had behavioral problems were shocked when they could not get their children to behave. Jessica is a psychologist and, before becoming a full-time mother, she counseled families with troubled children. Jessica's six-year-old son has trouble controlling his emotions and is aggressive with other children. These problems first manifested when he was four years old. She was absolutely dumbfounded by her son's defiance and aggression and, like Andrea, said that her efforts at perfection had fallen short. She said,

> [I have a lot of] training and I've read so many parenting books. And even early on, it seems like I was reading a parenting book a week. Not that that makes a good parent, but I *know* a lot of stuff. So I imagined I'd have these wonderfully behaved children because I just knew how to do it. And what a laugh. What a joke . . . I sometimes imagine the more perfect mother I'd be if I'd been given a child a little less challenging.

The disruption of maternal "perfection" is likely a class-specific phenomenon. The successful performance of intensive mothering requires time, money, and education.[2] When their children essentially blocked their maternal performances, the disruption was keenly felt among women who, like Andrea and Jessica, had the symbolic and material resources to thoroughly "prepare" for this particular enactment of motherhood.

Although children's problems undermined one set of images women had held about themselves as mothers, they sometimes presented women with new avenues for constructing valued identities. As noted in an earlier chapter, some mothers adopted professional presentations of self in order to evade mother-blame and secure desired resources during their interactions with medical and educational gatekeepers. Carol had wholeheartedly embraced professionalism, not just as an interactional strategy, but as an approach to "good" mothering. She explained, "I'm one of these professional mothers who's on a mission here to make her son the best that he can be. . . . I'm really trying to be as professional as I can about learning about my child's disability and how to help him." Indeed, women such as Carol revised their definitions of "good mothering" to focus on advocacy carework and the development of "expertise."

Children's problems did not pose as great a threat to men's identities as "good fathers." On the contrary, greater involvement in children's daily lives—often a necessity for fathers, as I discussed in Chapter 3—gave some men a sense of accomplishment and pride that they might not otherwise have had. When Jason talked about himself as a father, for example, he highlighted his participation in therapy for his six-year-old son, diagnosed with autism at eighteen months old. Jason's greater involvement in his children's lives was partly facilitated by a divorce, but, as he explains, his son's "parent-driven" therapy also encouraged a high level of engagement.

> I have a parent training class I go to once every two weeks . . . because a lot of this is very parent-driven . . . and I just . . . I feel more involved. You know, recently I've been the one to kind of like do the groundwork. I'd heard about a karate program that sort of specializes and works with special needs kids, and I've kind of done the legwork to get him set up in that. And so from that perspective, [the divorce has] been great. I feel a lot more involved than I was prior to our separation. And um, quite frankly it's more rewarding.

The expansion of carework related to children's problems significantly altered some parents' respective commitments to family and paid work. Research in the sociology of family demonstrates how changing life circumstances can disrupt a person's work-life trajectory, turning them toward or away from family life.[3] "Extreme contingencies," like a family member's illness or the sudden loss of high-quality childcare, can thrust career-committed women out of full-time employment and more fully into domestic work.[4] Personal circumstances can intersect with structural conditions to drastically shift men's trajectories as well. For example, even fathers who set out with the intention of becoming the family's "breadwinner" can veer toward domesticity in the wake of unemployment or blocked mobility in the labor force.[5] Among the parents I interviewed, children's problems tended to increase the importance of childrearing among men and women alike and, especially for women, diminish the importance of career advancement.

Relinquishing employment, for the parents who did so, meant letting go of what had been a pivotal feature of their life histories. Kathy, for example, tried to maintain her full-time job after her infant son (now six years old) was diagnosed with cerebral palsy, but it eventually become untenable. She said, "I think the toughest thing was realizing I had to quit my job. That was hard. I mean, I was at the point I was ready to . . . but it was just the fact of I've always had a job. I've never not worked. So that was a struggle for me." In all but two cases, it was women, not men, who left paid labor or reduced their employment hours to meet the demands of childrearing. In most cases, this gendered division of labor appeared to be taken-for-granted. In other cases, women made less money or had more flexible hours than their spouses, so the decision seemed practical. When men left their jobs to become stay-at-home fathers, it was due to a rare alignment of events. For example, Bill was in the midst of changing jobs and moving out of state with his family when his infant son (now sixteen years old) began having seizures. He and his wife decided not to move, and, since Bill was temporarily unemployed, he became a stay-at-home dad. He recalled how difficult that transition was.

> [I was] basically depressed. Couldn't do a whole lot. Felt sorry for myself, felt sorry for my son. Couldn't get motivated. It was tough to try and find a job. Just moped around a lot. My son wasn't in day care at the time. So I was the primary caregiver . . . while my wife worked. She had a good job, she had the benefits. So you know, it would definitely be a dumb decision to make her stay home while I went out and looked for a job. That didn't make sense because we needed the benefits. That was too important . . . [So I just became] Mr. Mom.

Most parents talked about the interruption of their career trajectories with a mix of grief and gratitude. They missed their previous positions and aspirations but had learned to see their carework as meaningful and valuable. When I interviewed Bill, some fifteen years after he had become "Mr. Mom," he was working part-time at a non-profit agency, providing resources to the family members of children with special needs. He had remained his son's primary caregiver and said he was quite happy with his part-time employment, despite its low pay: "I'm working here, and I love working here, this is one of the best jobs I've ever had. But I don't have the number of hours that I'm used to, I'm not working forty. I'm not working at the same salary that I had before. I don't have the same benefit package that I had before. It hurts financially. But we take it all and put it all together, I'm a happier person." Sarah had revised her narrative in a similar fashion. Sarah's thirteen-year-old biological son was diagnosed with cerebral palsy at birth and is severely disabled. When I asked her if it had been difficult to leave the workforce in order to care for him, she talked at first about grieving the loss of her career.

> It's hard to think about possibilities in the future because [my son] is a big limitation. And my decision to care for him is a big limitation . . . I do [wonder], will I have some time maybe in ten years from now? Or at some point, I'll be able to maybe go and do something, some career . . . I have that desire still . . . but I honestly have little hope. . . . I read in a newspaper, I've seen pictures of businesswomen, or . . . different women doing different things. And I feel sad that, "Oh, I can't do that." You know? But [I'm] not really resentful anymore. Just sad . . . that's part of the grief.

Later in the interview, however, Sarah talked about the importance of her caregiving and the sense of purpose that it has given her. "I really got to the point where, 'Yes, I'm [a stay-at-home mother]. Out of love for [my son],' and . . . it's a privilege. It's a joy. . . . It's the sense of purpose that I have that's greater than I've ever had."

The disruption of parents' career trajectories was not simply a matter of leaving the workforce or reducing employment hours, however. Children's problems sometimes meant that whoever took the role of primary earner faced a new set of pressures. Tim turned down an attractive job offer, for example, because it required moving to a different area.

> One of the biggest ways that [James'] disability impacted us as a family were in a number of my career decisions. And some job opportunities that I had to say no to because it would have been too hard on the family. So I think there's probably a real good chance that we would be somewhere else doing something else—at least I would for a living—if we hadn't been so incredibly sensitive to not wanting to disrupt [our son] and [our son's] life.

Tim's wife's decision not to return to the workforce also rendered Tim vulnerable. Because he was the sole earner, he could not take risks at work:

> I've been in some job situations over the years where I quite frankly probably put up with a lot more garbage and lousy treatment from employers than I would have put up with if I felt I had more options. But there were many times when I would say, "Well, I can't really stand up for myself in this situation because [Eve] is home with [James], I'm the sole provider, I can't afford to lose this job, I've just gotta sit here and take it because [my family] is more important than my own ego or my own pride."

Patty felt stuck, like Tim, but for different reasons. Her husband had been a graduate student when their son, fifteen months old at the time, was diagnosed with autism. Because Patty was working forty hours a week and her job afforded health benefits, her husband stayed at home to facilitate their son's in-home therapeutic program. He eventually became a stay-at-home father. Patty's son is now thirteen, and she feels guilty for not spending more time at home. She briefly considered working part-time so that she and her husband could share responsibilities, but it simply did not make sense for her to leave her managerial position.

> The full time job was so much better than what the two part time jobs could do . . . and then the benefit issue you know? By my being a manager I had a lot more flexibility. . . . I had in many ways achieved a great deal of flexibility, and [my husband] knew that and didn't really want me to give that up. And the fact that what I could make was more than what we could make as two part-time earners.

Thus, even fully-employed parents like Tim and Patty experienced a shift in their orientation to paid work and family obligation. In cases like theirs, children's problems limited their flexibility and placed even greater importance on maintaining a steady income and health benefits.

Children's problems also interrupted parents' biographical narratives by transforming the anticipated temporal dimensions of parenthood. With few exceptions, parenthood is a permanent identity; we do not readily exit the roles of mother and father like we do those of "tourist" or "college student."[6] However, we do expect the *demands* of parenthood to diminish over time. The performance of "intensive parenting," which requires so much money, time, and energy, is thought to be a time-sensitive endeavor with a distinct endpoint: children's entry into adulthood.[7] To the extent that children's problems prevented them from becoming fully independent, parents could no longer look forward to this exit, at least not automatically. The loss of an imagined future was quite salient for the parents of children with intractable problems. Jen and Carl's thirteen-year-old adopted daughter was diagnosed with an attachment disorder when she was a toddler, and their eight-year-old adopted daughter was diagnosed as having fetal alcohol effects. Jen commented,

> I mean, one thing that's a big tough thing for us and many parents who are, have special needs kids is that you don't get that, "You're free at eighteen thing." That's a big deal. How we see our future has had to [alter] . . . and that's mindboggling. 'Cause you kind of have a plan of your life, you know. You finish your school, you get your career in gear. You marry, you have your children. You're done having your children, they're independent, they're off, and you have your retirement and your traveling. Huh-uh. We might have this child all the time.

The disruption of parents' imagined futures included the relationships they envisioned developing with their adult children. Valerie reflected on her relationship with her own mother and how different it is from the type of relationship she will be able to have with her eleven-year-old daughter, diagnosed with autism when she was five.

> You asked, you know, what kinds of things have I had to give up. One thing that has come to mind in the last few years is . . . I have a good relationship with my mom. And it's almost like it became, like, a girlfriend kind of relationship over the years. And we love to get together and have lunch and go shopping or spend a day scrapbooking or whatever. And that kind of thing . . . I'm not gonna have that kind of relationship with [my daughter] . . . it doesn't mean we wouldn't enjoy spending the day together, but there wouldn't be a lot of, you know, chatting and

gossiping and shopping and those kinds of things. I mean . . . it's gonna be a different kind of thing.

For some parents, children's problems had implications for narratives of self that reached far beyond the spheres of family or employment. Several of the birth parents I interviewed talked about themselves as suffering from the same "problems" that their children had. They believed they had passed down to their children problematic genetic traits, tendencies, and predispositions. In many cases, it was only *after* parents came to view children as having "significant problems" that these notions of self emerged. Keith, whose eleven-year-old daughter was diagnosed with autism when she was five, is a practicing lawyer with seemingly good social skills; he said that his daughter's autism has caused him to reconsider his own childhood quirkiness.

> It's funny to have an autistic child because my childhood was a little odd. I was always kind of an odd kid. And um, now having an autistic child, I can go back and think, "Oh, I probably had a little autism going on myself" (laughs). Probably still do. [. . .] I recognize that some of the genetics of this are clearly through me and my family . . . and like I said, I recognize now, looking back through the prism of [our daughter] on my childhood, I recognize that I must have come off as more than a little odd to a lot of people. In sort of a similar way. And so I recognize that I made some contributions to this (laughs) . . . that's not a problem for me to recognize.

Like Keith, some parents made tenuous, off-handed connections between their own characteristics and children's problems. However, two parents whose children were diagnosed with attention deficit/hyperactivity disorder went on to receive diagnoses themselves. Peg, whose sixteen-year-old son was diagnosed with ADHD when he was eight, explained,

> I have ADD, I've been diagnosed. My father . . . died before adult diagnosis was really available, but he had multiple and compounding problems, undiagnosed, untreated ADD, I think. . . . ADD runs in the family. Learning disabilities run in the family. . . . I suspected I had ADD many years before I got tested . . . [my son] was diagnosed before I was. And that's not unusual.

Mike, whose eight-year-old son was diagnosed with attention deficit disorder when he was five, sought an evaluation for himself at his wife's encouragement. Like Peg, he came to view himself as having the disorder after his son was diagnosed.

Just as an aside, we knew that there's a genetic component to ADD/ADHD . . . so then at age forty-plus, you get diagnosed with it yourself. Then it's a whole new ball of wax! . . . My wife, being the good researcher she is (laughs), she just would notice my response to some things. Keeping track or not keeping track of things. Plus the fact that we noticed a genetic component . . . and I had kind of been assessing, "Well, maybe there's something to this." And so I said, "Well, it's better to know than not know, so let's rule it out." So I did some testing . . . and "Yep. Okay."

Among the parents in this study, fathers were more likely than mothers to talk about themselves as the genetic culprits of children's problems. As Mike's comments illustrate, wives may have played a key role in the construction these narratives. Mothers whose children suffered from autism, attention deficit disorder, or alcoholism often said that their husbands (or, in a few cases, former husbands) were the genetic sources of their children's problems. Monica, for example, believed that her ex-husband, Jason—who did not strike me as autistic when I interviewed him beforehand—has an undiagnosed autism spectrum disorder. Jason and Monica's six-year-old son was diagnosed with autism when he was eighteen months old. Monica said,

I'm sure [my ex-husband] is on the spectrum. I'm sure he's on the autistic spectrum. His mom and I had a frank discussion after we separated and his mom said if her husband were diagnosed today, he'd be on the spectrum. These are things you don't know. They ask you those questions, and you're like "No, there's no predisposition." You know, "No, everybody's fine," and then you start learning, and it's like, "Holy shit . . . this make sense now."

When I prompted Monica to discuss what she viewed as the signs and symptoms of her ex-husband's problem, she explained,

He eats the same thing everyday for breakfast, he eats the same thing everyday for lunch. He is very methodical in his thinking . . . he's a system's analyst, that doesn't say much. He is very regimented and any time spontaneity was thrown his way he gets absolutely angry. I mean, it's like you're fuckin' with his world . . . [in his childhood] he really had no sympathy, no feeling of empathy . . . you could not have a negative thought or feeling, he didn't know what to do with it . . . there were other things . . . [he is] very cerebral, just no social skills . . . .

How this pattern of interactions between mothers and fathers unfolded is not entirely clear from these data, though it is likely tied to women's roles as "researchers" and their efforts to manage mother-blame.

As illustrated here, children's problems often transformed how parents talked about themselves as mothers and fathers, as professionals, and as persons in general. As parents changed, so did their sense of themselves in relationship to a broader community of ostensibly "normal," middle-class people.

SEPARATION FROM THE MIDDLE-CLASS "MAINSTREAM"

The story of Seymour Levov, the main character of Philip Roth's novel *American Pastoral*, is a pointed illustration of how children's successes and failures bear symbolically upon their parents' status as belonging to the American middle-class.[8] Handsome, popular, and athletic, Levov sheds his Jewish identity, marries a former beauty queen, buys a lovely home in the countryside, and takes over his father's lucrative glove factory. He epitomizes the American dream. Levov's daughter Merry, however, suffers from a speech impediment, a stutter that persists despite extensive therapy and his wife's best efforts. As Merry approaches adolescence in the 1970s, she becomes overweight and confrontational. She joins the anti-war movement, and, when she kills an innocent man by detonating a bomb at the local post office, Levov's life falls apart. His beautiful wife suffers a nervous breakdown, they both have extramarital affairs, and, in the wake of race riots, Levov is forced to close his father's factory. In this story, Merry's fall from grace represents more than just her family's demise; it symbolizes the lost hopes of an entire generation and the death of the "American mythic ideal."[9] It is appropriate that Roth chose to use a child's problems as the catalyst for Levov's tragedy. Successful children are markers of belonging to the American middle-class. Childbearing itself is thought to be an integral part of the "good life," what it means to become an adult and to have one's own family.[10] Though parenthood is not the moral imperative that it was during the pro-natalist 1950s and '60s, most people still define the "ideal family" as one that includes children.[11]

Thus, the disruption of parents' selves in the wake of children's problems involved, at a fundamental level, a loss of status. Children's problems aligned participants and their families with low-status groups. For example, Claire, whose nine-year-old son was diagnosed with autism when he was three, commented that low-status mothers were more likely than middle-class white mothers to encourage their children to befriend her autistic son. She said,

> The people who are kind and actually encourage [their kids] to be friends with [my son] are very often poor people, single moms, immigrants. The mothers, particularly at the school, the white, upper-middle class mothers, the volunteers, the ones that are always organizing the fundraisers and such, inevitably will prevent friendship between their kids and my kid.

Phil, who was worried that other parents would blame him for his son's involvement in selling drugs, associated his son's deviance with poor, non-white youth. Phil's seventeen-year-old son began using and selling drugs three years ago. He was diagnosed with ADHD when he was in the sixth-grade and has also been in trouble for fighting. Phil talked at length about how his son's friends behave like members of an inner city gang, despite being white and middle-class.

> They're just wannabes . . . it was like, "Do you realize how ridiculous you look if you're trying to come over as being tough?" . . . but it was part of the persona that apparently [our son] wanted. And that's more concerning in some senses. Because you know, so-called gangs are infesting even towns like [ours] . . . it goes beyond just the drug use. . . . [We live in] a town of about fifty thousand. . . . I would say [it's] middle class . . . our houses are the average track houses, six hundred, six hundred and fifty thousand. So it's not cheap. I don't want to make this ethnic or cultural, but there's been a big infusion of Latinos . . . and there are lower rent apartments and things of that nature. And I think that's brought a little bit of the drug culture.

Special education also brought children into contact with stigmatized others. Lauren, though eager to secure biomedical labels for her twin ten-year-old adopted daughters' problems, fought tirelessly to keep them in mainstream classrooms. The girls were identified as having pervasive developmental delays when they were three. Lauren explained,

> From the very beginning the school has wanted [my daughters] to go into a special day class, and I've always objected. After two years of objecting to it, they said, "Why don't you just go visit a class and tell me what you think." And I went and visited two special day classes and went literally screaming and said, "I'll never do that. I'll never put my kids in that" . . . there were kids that should be potty trained that aren't. And you can tell. You can smell them.

As evinced here, stigma is not just a matter of negative labeling but also involves downward movement in the social hierarchy.[12] In light of this status loss, parents talked about themselves in opposition to what they imagined were "normal," middle-class families. Kathy, whose six-year-old son had been diagnosed with cerebral palsy when he was an infant, said, "The first year was just a real emotional time for me. I would just cry at nothing. . . . I'd be in the shower and I'd start bawling. And now that I look back on it, I think it was just my emotional feelings of dealing with the fact that I don't have a normal [life]." "Normalcy" became shorthand for the imagined lives parents had lost: careers, holidays, travel, retirement plans, and other deeply rooted assumptions about the "well-lived life." Tim, whose seventeen-year-old son has Fragile X syndrome (a genetic condition that became evident when the boy was a toddler), described the "ordinary" people who populate his middle-class neighborhood as occupying a different world, one that he and Eve no longer have access to.

> You see other people spending time with their kids in various things . . . saying, "Hey, you want to come see our kid's play tonight?" or you know, "Our child made the finals in the drama club," or who knows what? And you just can't relate to any of that. You can't participate in any of that because it's not your world.

Even parents whose children had fewer limitations defined themselves in opposition to "everybody" else. Sarah's seventeen-year-old stepson, who has had drug and alcohol problems since he was fifteen, was a senior in high school and had no plans following graduation. She was stung by how this separated her family from others in their affluent, highly educated community.

> Everybody asks, "Oh, what's gonna happen after high school?" And it's painful! . . . I get emails from the senior class parent group, and every day . . . "What are the seniors doing?" They're going to the career center. And they're thinking about this, and college, and la la la. And we're just . . . we're not in that same situation.

These comments demonstrate how, beyond specific challenges to men's and women's identities, the disruption stemming from children's problems led parents to place themselves outside the imagined American "mainstream." Judy's twenty-five-year-old son was diagnosed with attention deficit disorder in the sixth-grade. In Judy's words, having a problem child was just not commensurate with being a "nice" family.

JUDY: [Sometimes Jason] would get angry and rush out of the house. Slam the door. There was a lot of noise at our house. We're nice people, but there was a lot of noise sometimes. That was a sanity quotient for me. I wanted to stay a nice people. It was important to me to be a nice people.
ARA: Tell me what you mean by it.
JUDY: It meant that we were still nice, ordinary people in that we didn't have big horrible bad dysfunctional problems . . . at times, [Jason] and this ADD factor were pushing me off that desire to be a normal, ordinary, nice people.

This exchange with Judy calls to mind one of Erving Goffman's most famous quotes regarding the nature of stigma and "normalcy": "in an important sense there is only one complete unblushing male in America: a young, married, white, urban, northern, heterosexual Protestant father of college education, fully employed, of good complexion, weight, and height, and a recent record in sports."[13] Much has changed since the publication of *Stigma* in 1963, and the ostensibly "normal" or "ideal" constellation of identities has no doubt shifted. Nonetheless, the critique implicit in this quote remains just as poignant today as it was fifty years ago: no one is always or altogether "normal." Yet, the idea of "ordinary" loomed large in parents' imaginations as they struggled to make sense of the distance between the lives that they had imagined for themselves and the lives that they were living. As I later discuss, "normalcy" became the backdrop against which they constructed new selves.

Parents' hierarchical locations likely increased the magnitude of their sorrows because, unlike so many people in the United States, they had the symbolic and material resources necessary for the attainment of "the good life." The fact that several parents said that children's problems were the greatest challenges they had ever faced speaks not just to the priceless nature of children in the late-modern West and the central place of "healthy" children in American family life, but also to the comparatively privileged biographies of the parents in this study. When people expect the world to unfold according to the principles of rationality, tragedies pose a much greater threat to their sense of security and well-being. In other words, those that expect life to follow a "logical" sequence that adheres to a particular set of norms cannot easily make sense of suffering.[14] By and large, the men and women I interviewed were accustomed to things going *as planned*; most had college educations, steady jobs, and homes of their own. For many of these parents, children's problems were a profound first lesson in life's irrationality. That children's problems often stood in such stark contrast to the rest of parents' biographies made trouble seem unfamiliar and difficult to bear.

DEGREES OF ANOMIE

Parents' isolation, sense of otherness, and feelings of grief, guilt, and anxiety are best understood not as psychological problems, but as expressions of anomie. Anomie is traditionally defined as a state of "normlessness," or a breakdown of the rules that govern action and interaction. For Émile Durkheim, anomie was a byproduct of rapid modernization in the West; he argued that the transition from rural to urban society created a temporary period of normlessness as traditional ways of life declined and organic solidarity came to replace mechanical solidarity.[15] Robert Merton in contrast, argued that anomie is created by an imbalance of culture and structure in the United States; when people universally value economic success but are not universally afforded opportunities to become economically successful, anomie is the result.[16] Despite its theoretical importance in sociology, anomie is not a well-defined concept, and Merton's use of the term differed from Durkheim's in a number of important ways.[17] For example, Iain Wilkinson argues that Durkheim was more concerned with the social psychology of human suffering than Merton's revision of anomie suggests.

> Stjipan Mestrovic and Helene Brown (1985) argue that Robert Merton's (1957) "bland" and "essentially painless" interpretation of anomie as "normlessness" fails to convey the passionate emphasis upon the qualitative experience of social injustice evoked by Durkheim's original use of the term. . . . They contend that Durkheim always understood the meaning of anomie (and its synonym, *deregle-ment*) to refer not only to a lack of moral regulation in social life, but also to the inner feelings of pain and suffering that this is liable to engender.[18]

Peter Berger captures the subjective experience of anomie and offers a point of departure for thinking about parents' troubles in these terms.[19] As I explained in the introductory chapter, Berger views social order as imbuing life with meaning and protecting people from existential chaos. However, social order is always precarious because it is a human project requiring constant maintenance. This frailty becomes apparent when people are faced with "marginal situations," or moments when "definitions of reality—of the world, of others, and of self" are radically challenged.[20] Death, Berger argues, is the quintessential marginal experience because it "puts in question the taken-for-granted, 'business as usual' attitude in which one exists in everyday life."[21] If marginal experiences such as death are left unexplained, people begin to "see through" the social artifice and are exposed to the terror of meaningless. Berger explains,

> The primacy of the social objectivations of everyday life can retain its subjective plausibility only if it is constantly protected against terror. On the level of meaning, the institutional order represents a shield against terror. *To be anomic, therefore, means to be deprived of this shield and to be exposed, alone, to the onslaught of nightmare.* While the horror of aloneness is probably already given in the constitutional sociality of man, it manifests itself on the level of meaning in man's incapacity to sustain a meaningful existence in isolation from the nomic constructions of society. The symbolic universe shelters the individual from ultimate terror by bestowing ultimate legitimation upon the protective structures of the institutional order.[22]

Here Berger uses "anomie" in reference to the separation of individuals from socially constructed meanings held intact by social order. When used in this way, anomie is not just a state of normlessness, but also a state of meaninglessness.

For some of the parents in this study, children's problems constituted a marginal situation that led them to question long-held beliefs and taken-for-granted assumptions about their own lives and the world around them. For example, Tim, whose seventeen-year-old son was diagnosed with Fragile X syndrome as a toddler, commented on how his son's disabilities shook his religious beliefs.

> I'm a person of deep religious faith. At the time it caused me to really question and kind of get angry with God. "God, what are you doing here, I don't get this" [. . .]. I just didn't understand why this had happened and why it had been laid on us . . . when really traumatic things happen that you don't understand, you kind of go through this kind of soul-searching, "Why?" You know, "What does this all mean in the scheme of life?" And so it took me a while, I'm ashamed to admit. It took me a while to kind of get through that and stop being mad at God.

Sentiments like these were more common among parents whose children had severe, intractable problems. Mild learning disabilities, for example, did not result in the same level of existential questioning. However, most of the parents I interviewed described a fundamental shift in perspective as they struggled to make sense of their children's (and their own) departure from the perceived norm. Paula, whose eight-year-old son was diagnosed with attention deficit disorder when he was five, said that her experiences were not unlike those of parents whose children have traditional disabilities: "Helplessness, helplessness. I think it's a loss. You know, because I always pictured [my son] to be the captain of a Jesuit football team. And I doubt that's gonna happen . . . it's a different path that he's on. It's similar to a parent who thinks that they're gonna have a normal child and they have a Down Syndrome child . . . you know, you just have to re-adjust and re-evaluate. And grieve." Though her son's problems did not culminate in an existential crisis, Paula's need to "re-adjust" and "re-evaluate" illustrates how she, like Tim, must grapple with what her son's problems mean. Forced to relinquish the taken-for-granted assumptions about his future, as well as many of the expectations she had regarding motherhood, she must reorient how she makes sense of her son, herself, and her family in light of her son's ostensible departure from "normal."

As defined by the theorists cited earlier, anomie refers to an extreme disconnection of the person from social order. For Durkheim and Merton, this disconnection results in suicide or crime. For Berger, it gives way to feelings of "terror." However, the concept of anomie is also useful for theorizing the less dramatic experiences of disconnection described by the parents in this study. As I have illustrated, the view that children had "serious problems" initiated a wave of disruption that rippled throughout parents' lives. The micro-social order that served to maintain parents' sense that everything was "okay" was now in flux. As a consequence, parents came to feel unanchored, no longer sure of their place in social life and no longer confident that they had somewhere to belong. Parents' subjective experiences of anomie—anxiety, sadness, loneliness—varied by degree but stemmed from the same basic dynamics of trouble.

On one hand, most of the parents I interviewed were unable to return to their former selves or to the lives they had imagined living. On the other hand, some had been able to, in Paula's words, "re-adjust" and "re-evaluate" so that things made sense again, life was no longer so chaotic, and a sense of belonging was regained. There were a few avenues that allowed parents to restore narrative continuity. Trying to correct children's problems—or to "normalize" their conduct—was the first path taken by most parents, though, as I have suggested, this strategy had uneven results and generated its own kind of trouble. In the end, some parents found solace in their relationships with other troubled parents. While some support groups had a strong culture of advocacy care and further encouraged mothers' remedial efforts, most also provided sense-making narratives and new relationships that allowed parents to re-anchor themselves to social life. Despite narratives of healing and uplift, though, not all parents participated in support groups or told stories that featured "acceptance" or "closure." Indeed, some of the men and women I interviewed suffered daily and simply "made do."

MEDICALIZATION AND "NORMALIZATION"

As I have argued, biomedical accounts of children's conditions and behaviors had the potential to mitigate parents' experiences of stigma but were more effective in doing so when they were widely accepted. When people questioned the legitimacy of medical labels and, for example, mothers had to fight for special educational accommodations, the effects of stigma could be more salient, rather than less. Nonetheless, some mothers reported that their efforts to find suitable diagnoses and treatments for children's problems did help to "normalize" their conditions or behaviors, and, in turn, allowed parents to maintain the "restitution narrative"[23] I discussed in Chapter 3. These parents held strongly to the notion that their children had been sick but that medical science had rendered them well again. For example, Jessica's six-year-old son had been so aggressive with other children that, when he was four years old, he was nearly expelled from his preschool. Several months after our interview, Jessica sent me an email that said, "Just for your information, [our son] is doing GREAT! He started some antidepressants that have helped him immensely. Needless to say, the family is also doing great as a result." Parents' efforts to treat invisible disabilities were rarely so successful, but as Jessica's comments suggest, pharmaceutical interventions and behavioral therapies did sometimes improve children's conduct and parents' situations.

As demonstrated by Andrea's story described earlier, parents' investment in therapeutic boarding schools designed to rehabilitate rebellious or drug addicted teenagers yielded inconsistent results. Seth and Rhonda, whose daughter began abusing drugs and ran away from home when she was fourteen, reported the most success with this form of treatment (now nineteen, their daughter was sober and living at home). However, even these parents were unsure about the program's effectiveness, and the theme of restitution did not feature as strongly in their narratives.

SETH: [Our daughter] works with me now. . . . She's there everyday, she's great. She's an asset. She's living with us, everything is good . . . and it's been good since the day she came home. . . . I don't know anyone else [in her program] who had that experience . . . so I don't know how much I can say, "Yeah, therapeutic boarding school is a great thing." It might have just been that she needed that time away from [here], and it wouldn't have mattered where she was. Because I see a lot of these kids who went through the same exact program, and as soon as they came back, they went right back into it. So . . . who knows?

RHONDA: And even with, you know, sort of rave reviews with the staff, and all of that . . . [our daughter] still struggles with her issues.

It was more common for the parents of delinquent adolescents to live in a state of uncertainty, continuously vacillating between feelings of hope and despair.

Contrary to finding the panacea they had hoped for, a number of mothers said that, in retrospect, their intensive efforts to procure medical and educational resources had prolonged their troubles. As I have explained, the sheer difficulty of making and keeping appointments, preparing for meetings, and managing their emotions during interactions with bureaucratic gatekeepers prevented some mothers from fully experiencing the sadness and loss associated with their children's problems. Indeed, many parents eventually abandoned their efforts to "normalize" children's conduct. Their troubles were sometimes mitigated, instead, through their alignment with fellow-sufferers.

ALIGNING WITH FELLOW-SUFFERERS

Suffering offers opportunities for solidarity.[24] Among the men and women I interviewed, connecting to other parents in trouble operated in this way. Some participants regained a sense of belonging through their identification with parents whose children have problems. When they talked about how children's problems had changed them, they talked not only about their separation from the "mainstream," but their newfound membership in an imagined community of "outsiders." Claire, whose nine-year-old son was diagnosed with autism when he was three, volunteers with an autism advocacy group and is well-networked with parents of children with special needs. She said,

> I think that when you have a kid with special needs, there's a major shift in the way you see life. And you see yourself as belonging to a group of people who sees the world differently. . . . You all the sudden align yourself with people who know a certain kind of pain, who have a certain kind of world view, you know? . . . There's a certain life experience that bonds you because you understand something. So I feel this affinity to other parents that have kids with special needs.

Similarly, one of the most salient parts of Steve and Marie's visit to their daughter's therapeutic boarding school was listening to the gut-wrenching stories of other parents. Six months prior to our interview, Steve and Marie discovered that their seventeen-year-old daughter is a cocaine addict.

STEVE: Boy, [Marie] and I, when we flew home on that plane from that first visit when it was the parents' seminar thing, I mean, we looked at each other and said, "My god. Everybody's got a story." I mean, what an eye opener that was! . . . I mean, we've been through the mill . . . [but] it's nothing compared to some of these multi-year, two- and three-year battles with some of these kids.

MARIE: We felt fortunate.

STEVE: The expressions on some of these parents that have been fighting this multi-year battle . . . it's a mind-boggling experience. Uh, just the look of—I don't want to say desperation—but just *tiredness*. Just the tiredness. That woman that was in my group, that little gal from Petaluma that I really liked?

MARIE: Uh-huh.

STEVE: God, she was a little bitty thing. Petaluma, California. Uh, she was in my small group of five or six. She was the most soft-spoken, nicest woman (begins to cry). She reminded me of my mother (pauses to cry). She [had a] long battle with this kid . . .

MARIE: Yeah, no, she was a nice lady.

STEVE: You know, [and she said], "I'm still trying, I'm still fighting," you know? And you just, your heart goes out to 'em.

By realizing that "everybody's got a story," Steve and Marie are able to rewrite their own narrative. They've been "through the mill," yes, but relative to many parents, they're "fortunate." Their identification with "fellow sufferers"[25] provided a vantage point from which they could talk about empathy and gratitude instead of isolation and despair.

Gratitude often emerged from this realignment because, as Steve and Marie's comments suggest, participants encountered families whose troubles seemed greater than their own. Lauren, whose ten-year-old adopted daughters have pervasive developmental delays, commented, "I do walk away [from conversations with other parents] going, 'Oh my god, I have no problems. What am I getting upset for? I am so lucky!' Because families are dealing with *so* much." In the most concrete sense, support groups helped parents to fend off isolation when their children's problems had disrupted their relationships with family members and close friends. Kathy, whose six-year-old son was diagnosed with cerebral palsy before his first birthday, said that it was difficult to talk about her son's problems with her usual group of friends, but she found solace in a local support group.

> I had [other] friends, but they were always like, "Oh, [your son] is fine." So I just wouldn't talk to them. . . . "You don't get it" (laughs). "He's not fine" (laughs). You know? It's a totally different . . . it's like, well they're not gonna understand anyway because their kids are normal. You know, they're not struggling with these kinds of things, so it's gonna be not the same for them . . . [in my town] there's a support group for parents with special needs kids . . . and I started attending that . . . and so that was helpful because then I could talk to those parents and they went through the same things I did.

Perhaps most importantly, support and advocacy networks provided some parents with a new language for making sense of their children's problems. For example, the mothers of children with invisible disabilities learned how to wield biomedical accounts, not by visiting doctors, but by becoming involved in support and advocacy networks. Grace, whose seventeen-year-old adopted daughter was diagnosed with attention deficit disorder in the sixth-grade and also suffers from depression, was a member of an organization designed to support people with ADD. In the course of attending meetings, she adopted the rhetoric used by experts who defend the legitimacy of ADD as a medical diagnosis. She commented, for example,

> People think [children] are over-medicated or over-diagnosed. . . . Doctor Edward Hallowell, he did *Driven to Distraction*, and he's been at a lot of [our] conferences. And he's gone even on the Today Show . . . [he says] it's really *under-diagnosed* because basically they think three to five percent of children have it. And there's only been one percent diagnosed.

Though not always able to mitigate "enacted stigma," or stigma that is manifest in interaction, by deploying medical labels, parents like Grace used biomedical accounts to avoid internalizing people's negative impressions.[26]

As mentioned in the previous chapter, support groups also offered parents a vocabulary for talking about the pain of loss. I had contacted eight participants through "The Parent Share," a local organization designed to help parents whose children have special needs.[27] Most of these parents employed a popular grief discourse loosely premised on Elizabeth Kübler-Ross's stage model.[28] For example, Lauren, whose twin, ten-year-old adopted daughters have pervasive developmental delays, spontaneously broached the subject of grief during her interview, and she gave me a handout called titled "The 'Good' Grief Cycle." She explained,

> I don't know if you've run across this. There's a psychologist named Ken Moses, and they have videos. In fact, [The Parent Share] has a borrowing library that you're welcome to go use, [and they have] videos of Ken Moses. And this is what he talks about. The good grief cycle. And this is the cycle of families that have special-needs children. It's a circle for a reason. It's because you never get out of it.

The handout Lauren had given me featured a circle surrounded by the following words in clockwise order: shock, depression, denial, guilt, shame, isolation, panic, anger, bargaining, hope, acceptance. The words were listed again below the diagram, this time with brief definitions and explanations. Lauren went on to say, "Personally [I] did this. I was looking at it one day, and I said, You know, I always have hope, I have depression, I'm sure I have denial, I'm sure the professionals said, 'Boy, that's a parent in denial.' And I have panic. And I can be euphoric one minute and literally the next minute [I'm] scraping myself off the ground." As these comments suggest, Lauren borrowed terminology from a commonly shared grief discourse in order to articulate her feelings. It is possible that this discourse not only provided parents with the words to describe their emotions, but also played a role in generating new feelings. Lauren's remark that she is "sure" she has denial illustrates how parents may have worked to align their own experiences with discourse.

Support groups also encouraged parents to reframe children's "problems." This is exemplified by "Welcome to Holland," a widely-published piece mentioned by three parents whose children had developmental disabilities. The author likens having a child with disabilities to planning a vacation to Italy, only to discover, upon arrival, that one has landed in Holland instead. The narrative capitalizes on the critical orientation to disability as "difference," as illustrated in this excerpt:

> The important thing is that [Holland is not a] . . . horrible, disgusting, filthy place, full of pestilence, famine and disease. It's just a different place . . .

It's slower-paced than Italy, less flashy than Italy. But after you've been there for a while and you catch your breath, you look around . . . and you begin to notice that Holland has windmills . . . and Holland has tulips. Holland even has Rembrandts.

But everyone you know is busy coming and going from Italy . . . and they're all bragging about what a wonderful time they had there. And for the rest of your life, you will say "Yes, that's where I was supposed to go. That's what I had planned."

And the pain of that will never, ever, ever, ever go away . . . because the loss of that dream is a very very significant loss.

But . . . if you spend your life mourning the fact that you didn't get to Italy, you may never be free to enjoy the very special, the very lovely things . . . about Holland.[29]

"Welcome to Holland" suggests that, although grief is expected, there is still much to celebrate about having a child with special needs, and parents should not spend their lives in bereavement for the child they expected. A few parents echoed this sentiment. I interviewed Jen and Carl about their two adopted daughters, one of whom has an attachment disorder and the other of whom has fetal alcohol effects. Shortly before Jen described "Welcome to Holland," Carl said, "The rewards [of having children with special needs] come in ways that you can't really plan on and can't really expect . . . it's frustrating when, when *your* ideas about the ways that you think you want it may not happen, but there's other things that are very positive too, so [you have to] be open for new things."

Al-Anon promoted a very different framework for narrating children's "problems" and talking about sorrow. Rather than employing a grief discourse, Al-Anon emphasized the importance of taking care of oneself and not allowing one's life to be overcome by a child's alcohol or drug abuse. Deborah, whose twenty-six-year-old son has been an alcoholic since he was fifteen, recalled how Al-Anon meetings helped her manage the grief associated with her son's problems. She said,

[I was] going into meetings and sitting there and listening to people talk about what it was like and how they survived it. And [they were] just saying, "It'll be okay. It'll be okay. *You'll* be okay," you know? "Things may not be the way you want them to be, but *you will be* okay . . . ." [Without Al-Anon] I think I would be an absolute wreck. I know how bad I was . . . before I got into the program. . . . I was physically sick . . . emotionally, I was a wreck. I was anorexic. I didn't sleep.

While organizations like Parent Share encouraged parents to work through their grief by focusing on the positive aspects of parenting a child with disabilities, Al-Anon encouraged parents to manage their feelings by "letting go" of their attempts to control the behavior of their alcoholic or drug addicted children. Their underlying premise is that parents tend to enable children's destructive behavior by repeatedly trying to "fix" their problems and that by developing clearer emotional boundaries, parents will help their children and themselves. This "emotional distance" coping strategy seemed to provide some solace for parents who attended Al-Anon meetings.

MAKING SENSE AND MAKING DO

In studies of illness, a "quest narrative" is one that assumes there is something to be learned or gained from the experience of suffering.[30] Unlike the restitution narrative, which celebrates medical science, the quest narrative elevates the sufferer's own voice and focuses on his or her "journey" to find meaning in hardship. Some parents embraced such a narrative, focusing not only on what they had lost but also on what they had gained from children's problems. Theirs were narratives of silver linings and joy, despite great sorrow. For example, some parents of children with developmental disabilities said that they were grateful for not having to worry about the difficulties associated with "normal" adolescents. Valerie, whose eleven-year-old daughter had been diagnosed with autism at the age of five, explained,

> [My daughter] is eleven-years-old, and lately I find myself really appreciating her disability a lot because one great thing that's happening is that all of the girls around her are getting to that age where girls begin to hate themselves and feel ugly and worry about their weight, and all that just completely goes over [my daughter's] head. She's not concerned. She wears her little t-shirts and sweat pants, and she has very short hair . . . she thinks her body is great . . . she's not into boys, and she's not into any of the things that a lot of the girls her age are into. And so that I see as a real perk (laughs) . . . there's a lot of difficult things coming up in the next few years that she's not gonna probably get interested in.

In the case of gifted children and children with learning disabilities, parents linked their children's problems to more desirable attributes such as intelligence or creativity. Judy, whose twenty-five-year-old son was diagnosed with attention deficit disorder in the sixth-grade, commented,

> Usually [children with ADD] are bright. These kids are usually a little brighter than the average kid. I mean, it's not a bunch of dumb kids that have ADD. Oftentimes it's brighter ones. And then you also see where that ADD goes though in a positive light. I mean, look at Hollywood. Look at your famous authors, look at your scientists. I mean, look at these people who are outside

that box when it really really wasn't popular to be. Donald Trump, Ross Perot, I mean, these are all over-the-top guys.

Even parents whose children had drug and alcohol problems sometimes talked about silver linings in the midst of otherwise heartbreaking situations. For example, Steve and Marie, who discovered six months prior to our interview that their seventeen-year-old daughter was a cocaine addict, hoped that when all was said and done, their daughter would be a better person because of her battle with addiction.

STEVE: One of the positive byproducts of this whole process is we actually *believe*, anyway at this point, that we're . . . getting a better kid back than the one we sent, in a lot of different ways. Obviously one that's not on cocaine anymore. Uh, but on the emotional side and the character side . . .

MARIE: More mature.

STEVE: You know, we could fill two of [your recorders] with the changes and the growth that she's shown. You know, like [my wife] said, I wish I could shove some of that into her sisters up the line (laughs). You know?

MARIE: Or [have] every teenager go through some of this [therapy].

Many of the men and women I interviewed talked about parenting as a joyful experience, despite their troubles. When asked quite directly, all but a handful of parents said that they would do it all over again. Sarah knew during pregnancy that her child would have significant problems; her thirteen-year-old biological son was diagnosed with cerebral palsy at birth and is severely disabled. She said that although she could not have imagined the pain she would experience because of her son's disabilities, she does not regret her decision to have him. She explained,

I recently came up with the title for the book I end up writing about [my son], if I ever do . . . *Intangible Grief, Surprising Joy.* Something like that. You know, both sides are really intense. I'm just really surprised at how much joy there is, but also the depth of intangible grief. . . . [Later in the interview . . .] Honestly, most of the time, I would say the joys outweigh the pain.

The selves that emerged in narratives like these had greater wisdom and were more compassionate than parents' previous selves. Like Andrea, whose story I recounted in this chapter's introduction, some parents also said that children's troubles had made them better people. At different points in the past ten years, Amanda's fifteen-year-old son has been diagnosed with attention deficit/hyperactivity disorder, dyslexia, and bipolar disorder. Amanda commented,

"The difficulties have brought knowledge and understanding, and I think any difficulty with a child makes you less judgmental and more sensitive to other people. . . . [My son's] situation has made me so open-minded to other people and what's going on with them." Similarly, Tim, whose seventeen-year-old son was diagnosed with Fragile X syndrome when he was a toddler, talked at length about how his son's disabilities had made him a more compassionate person.

> I think I'm a deeper person—I mean, that's a real broad term—but I believe I have a better ability to relate to people who are in difficult circumstances. I think I have more sympathy for people who are down and out. And . . . even though I had an element of that in me because of my Christian faith from the beginning, I think I've really gotten more textured and layered and more nuanced in my ability to identify with people's problems and to sympathize with them, to be there for 'em, to really kind of be a shoulder to lean on. I think my ability to do that and to do it with the right heart has been improved because of my own experience. I mean, it's sort of the fellowship of suffering, if you will. You know, so I think that's made me a better person.

Again and again, parents underscored how children's problems developed their ability to empathize with others in trouble. This, like so many aspects of parents' troubles, should be understood in terms of parents' social locations and class-specific constructions of "normalcy." For example, Claire, whose nine-year-old son was diagnosed with autism when he was three, suggested that prior to the autism diagnosis she was just as oblivious as the upper-middle class mothers who discourage their children from befriending her son. Feeling as though she and her son are on the outside has transformed her, and, in turn, she views herself as a better mother and a better person.

> I wonder about myself before I got a diagnosis for [my son]. I mean, I see the world so differently now, and I think that people ought to encourage their children to invite the kid with a disability to a birthday party, etcetera. But that's just part of opening life up to their kid. And for manifesting your values. But I don't know whether I was like that [before], you know? I think I've become more compassionate too. . . . I see mothering now as being more about guiding your kids to be happy and empathetic, as opposed to playing the musical instrument and being a good athlete and getting them the best education, which is why we came [to this town]. I think that my values have shifted slightly, you know?

This quote from Claire makes explicit the relationship between social class, "normalcy," and the reconstruction of parents' selves in light of children's problems. Though parents longed to be "normal" at times and were devastated by their losses, the new selves they constructed depended on the foil of "normal," middle-class people. Claire no longer conceived of herself as belonging to a set of privileged parents who value musical talent, athleticism, and educational advancement. Her values, now focused on happiness and empathy, are a source of pride, not merely a reflection of stigmatization or loss.

Stories like Claire's had the quality of an "awakening" narrative; parents once were blind but could now "see the light."[31] The families around them were seemingly focused on competition, achievement, and the symbolic accouterments of middle-class American living. Some parents looked back at their personal histories and recognized that they, too, had cared about such things. However, their children's problems led them to reject those values, and they were happier for having done so. Lisa, the mother of two children with hyperinsulinism (one of whom sustained brain damage at birth), talked about garnering a sense of freedom to be herself, unencumbered by the pressure to be "normal."

> I think with kids, in society, there's such a demand to make your family this way and to be this way. And I think I've learned that time-outs don't work for all kids. You know, you have to take each child individually and take what works for them. Well I felt the pressure to do the normal thing, what everybody does with their kids, you know? My mother-in-law will call me and say, "Hey, so-and-so has this new computer . . . you need to have it for your five-year-old because she needs to learn." Well I'm like, "No, she doesn't have to have it. I don't care if so-and-so has it." You know, I can sit and play with her just as well. . . . I feel like I can just be myself and take [my kids] for who they are. And it's just easier.

Restitution and quest narratives are appealing to audiences because they imply some degree of triumph or closure. There is a danger in focusing on these elements of parents' stories, however. First, not all of the parents I interviewed spoke of gratitude, silver linings, or becoming better people. Illness narrative research demonstrates that some stories offer no promise of emotional growth or personal realization; instead, some narratives foreground the chaos and loss of control described in previous chapters.[32] Concluding with stories that foreground joy is, I fear, a disservice to those who did not strongly deploy the "journey" metaphor. Sometimes even well-networked parents who cherished their relationships to other mothers and fathers in trouble said that coming to terms with children's problems was an unending, painful endeavor. "Making do" was a central theme in those parents' narratives. Lauren, whose twin, ten-year-old daughters were diagnosed with developmental disabilities when they were three, made a brief comment that exemplifies this pattern: "What do you do? You just keep on keepin' on." Sometimes, there was nothing left to do other than persevere. Doug, together with his wife Sandra, was considering residential treatment for their thirteen-year-old adopted son. The couple had tried for more than a decade to remedy the boy's erratic, aggressive behavior and had recently started counseling for marital problems. Doug spoke very matter-of-factly about doing his best and bearing the ongoing frustration of not living the life he and Sandra had wanted: "Everybody wants what we want. But when you don't get it, then there's some level of frustration. When the path that you go on is chosen by virtue of the circumstances, then you don't have much control. You navigate it the best you can . . . those are your best choices . . . and you're aware of that . . . you're as comfortable as you can be, but you're still going to have a level of frustration." Unlike Claire, Tim, and other parents who talked about gaining wisdom and compassion, the most that Doug could say was that he was doing the best he could, given the circumstances. He is making do, much like Kathy, whose six-year-old son was diagnosed with cerebral palsy before his first birthday:

> There are times I am depressed. There are times when I don't want to get out of bed. There are times when I don't want to do it anymore. But I just do it. I don't know how I do it. Honestly I just know there's days I wake up and I don't want to, but I do (laughs).

In sum, some parents offered no "moral to the story" and talked, instead, about hauling themselves through each and every day, doing what needed to be done.

Through the conceptual lens of "family trouble," parents' sorrow, anxiety, and guilt are expressions of disconnection from social life. Family trouble may not always lead to anomie. However, when it involves the disruption of multiple, meaningful aspects of daily life, as it did among the parents in this study, it can generate feelings of otherness and throw into question taken-for-granted realities. For many parents, especially those who believed they had come out on the "other side" of family trouble, anomie was a temporary state. Even parents who were in the midst of family trouble worked to make sense of their children's problems, to reconnect themselves to larger communities of people, and to restore continuity to their narratives of self.

Framing parents' experiences in terms of "family trouble" highlights the social elements of their suffering. As I have demonstrated, understanding mothers' and fathers' inner turmoil requires more than knowledge of what occurred in their minds and bodies. It also demands an understanding of their place in relationship to specific and generalized others. Suffering may reside in individual psyches, but trouble is located in the social order. In the next and final chapter of this book, I examine the relevance of parents' experiences to other types of family-related disruption.

7 · FAMILY TROUBLE

C. Wright Mills's distinction between personal troubles and public issues is a cornerstone of sociological thought and remains, more than fifty years later, one of the most familiar ways of articulating the sociological perspective. In Mills's words,

> The sociological imagination enables its possessor to understand the larger historical scene in terms of its meaning for the inner life and the external career of a variety of individuals. It enables him to take into account how individuals, in the welter of their daily experience, often become falsely conscious of their social positions. Within that welter, the framework of modern society is sought, and within that framework the psychologies of a variety of men and women are formulated . . .
>
> Perhaps the most fruitful distinction with which the sociological imagination works is between "the personal troubles of milieu" and the "public issues of social structure." This distinction is an essential tool of the sociological imagination and a feature of all classic work in social science.[1]

Mills's argument implies a macro-social analysis, and as I argued in the introduction, parents' troubles cannot be understood in separation from the broad cultural meanings of children and family life among middle-class people in the late-Modern West. The sacralization of childhood and elevated significance of parenthood make fertile grounds for the type of family trouble these parents experienced. Children's problems were tremendously disruptive in the context of a culture that places children at the center of family life. Previous chapters further highlighted how parents' hierarchical positions, particularly with respect to gender and social class, but also in terms of race, shaped their personal woes. "Bright," "social," and "successful" children are markers of white, middle-class status and, for some, an integral part of what it means to be an "ordinary"

American. An ideology of intensive mothering reflects and reproduces historical legacies of gender inequality and renders mothers more susceptible than fathers to particular types of disruption related to children's problems.

Although historical, cultural, and hierarchical positions are important for understanding personal troubles, this in-depth look at parents' experiences illustrates how much we can gain by also looking at the micro-social dynamics of disruption. Routines and relationships are what connected parents' selves to the broader social contexts described here. In Mills's words, it is in the "welter of daily experience" that the self intersects with society. Exploring how children's problems disrupted the micro-social patterns of conduct that made up parents' taken-for-granted, everyday lives has been the focus and contribution of this book.

PARENTHOOD, SELF, AND SOCIETY

Mills encourages his readers to see how personal troubles are a product of broad economic and political contexts, but what are the mechanisms that link macro-social structures to what goes on in people's minds and bodies? It is one thing to recognize how parents' troubles are social issues. It is another thing to explain how, exactly, their thoughts and feelings are matters of social forces. The very idea might seem counterintuitive, given how our culture exalts individualism. When we think about society, if we think about it at all, we tend to see it as part of a broader environment that influences human conduct. In fact, this is how social psychologists trained in psychology often conceive of the relationship between societies and selves.[2] But to frame society as something that "affects" individual people is to miss one of the most basic contributions of the sociological perspective: human beings are social to the core. Social life does not "influence" the individual, it constitutes the individual.

The self is anchored in social space by the patterns of interaction that make up a person's everyday life.[3] For the people in this book, the roles of mother and father organized a wide swath of these patterns. Daily routines such as eating, sleeping, working, exercising, and relaxing; relationships with spouses, family members, and friends; encounters with acquaintances and strangers; narratives of self as "good" or "normal" mothers, fathers, professionals, and middle-class Americans, all of these social patterns were tied to parenthood and relied on having children whose conditions and behaviors remained broadly within the boundaries of people's shared expectations. When Seth said that his children are his life, he was not just speaking metaphorically. From an interactionist perspective, children are constitutive elements of these parents' selves.

As each chapter of this book illustrates, children's problems fractured the social scaffolding of parents' everyday lives. They unsettled the patterns of interaction that sustained parents' narratives, engendered biographical disruption and revision, and gave way to profound grief, guilt, and anxiety. These emotions contributed further to the disruption of daily life, leaving some parents to feel adrift from the social worlds they had previously identified with. The concept of "family trouble" captures the dynamic process of micro-social disruption and distress parents experienced. As a sensitizing concept, "family trouble" also helps to illuminate other cases of family-related disruption.

"FAMILY TROUBLE" AS A SENSITIZING CONCEPT

We tend to assume that families are venues for deep personal commitment and the development of salient identities. However, commitment to family-related roles is more variable than most people imagine, particularly as personal relationships have become increasingly flexible in the late-modern West. Social theorists argue that Western societies are undergoing a major transformation that has implications for the organization of personal life. Since the 1970s, especially, social life has become less fixed and relationships have become more fluid.[4] Phases of the life course—such as when people leave home, begin full-time employment, partner, and have children—are less predictable than they used to be, particularly for middle-class and affluent groups.[5] Furthermore, features of the social order that once served as primary venues of commitment—local communities and stable, long-term employment, for example—are on the decline. In tandem with these changes, "there is a growing ideological acceptance of individuals' rights to exercise fuller control over the ways they live their lives and the lifestyle choices they make."[6]

This has important, if somewhat paradoxical, ramifications for families. Sex, childbearing, and marriage—no longer linked tightly together—are seen more as matters of choice than of tradition. Ideologically, at least, late-modern families are premised not on legal or cultural directives, but on voluntary commitment, mutual affection, and self-fulfillment. On one hand, this means that personal investments in family life are not obligatory; it is more acceptable than ever before to remain unmarried, to be child-free, or to form one's deepest commitments outside the boundaries of traditionally-defined family life.[7] On the other hand, the expectations and possibilities for deep, personal investments in family life are also greater than ever before precisely because family relationships are considered voluntary. If people do get married, we expect them to love one another and even to conceive of themselves as "best friends."[8] If people do have children, we expect them to care very deeply about those children and to highly prioritize their health and well-being. Unlike previous eras in Western history, when families served explicitly political and economic functions, people see late-modern families first and foremost as venues for personal connection and personal fulfillment. Suffice to say, meaningful family commitments are not passé. Research suggests that, despite coming of age in an era of fluid relationships, most young men and women desire a family life that includes a committed partnership and children.[9]

This means that family-related disruption can be incredibly destabilizing.[10] Just as children's problems upended parents' lives, events such as death, illness, separation, and divorce can interrupt patterns of interaction between family members, threaten salient notions of self, and spill over into other spheres of interaction. Sociologists have long studied the social psychological ramifications of such events.[11] However, most situate their work within problem-specific bodies of literature and do not build on one another's research. As a result, we lack a shared framework for conceptualizing the personal troubles that stem from the disruption of family interaction. The sensitizing concept of "family trouble," defined in this book as any upheaval in family members' interactions that threatens salient aspects of self and results in intrapersonal turmoil, offers a point of departure for thinking about ostensibly disparate cases in generic sociological terms.

The lens of "family trouble," for example, illuminates striking parallels between relationship dissolution and having a child with significant problems. Like the participants in this study, couples on the precipice of separation or divorce experience a period of ambiguity. People come to see their relationships as "problematic" in the course of social interaction; trouble emerges slowly and indeterminately as people nurture new identities and share their dissatisfaction with sympathetic family members and friends.[12] Relationship dissolution is also characterized by the disruption of routine; efforts to salvage the relationship require time and energy, and separation is so time-consuming that people sometimes wait for a break in their schedules before initiating the break.[13] Like the family trouble associated with children's problems, relationship dissolution spills over into other relationships as friends and family members align with one spouse or the other.[14] Furthermore, each member of the couple must reorganize the roles and identities that had been tied to the relationship; when couples with children separate, for example, their performances of motherhood and fatherhood shift dramatically.[15] Finally, the social disruption stemming from separation and divorce results in cognitive and emotional turmoil. People "may have feelings of distress, depression, and anxiety, and they may display the actions that can accompany emotionally upsetting states, such as drinking and bodily responses in the form of physical symptoms."[16]

Anomie characterizes family troubles of all kinds. Across different types of disruption, scholars describe an experience of feeling adrift or unanchored. This is illustrated clearly in Debra Umberson's study of how adults experience and cope with losing a parent.

The crisis [stemming from a parent's death] can result in high levels of psychological distress, increased risk for depression, impaired physical health, or increased
alcohol consumption. . . . Most adults are surprised by the intensity and per-
sistence of their reactions, and are thrown off balance when their distress fuels
changes in their interpersonal relationships, behaviors, social roles, and even in
the ways in which they view themselves.[17]

The same was once true of long-distance marriages. Thirty years ago, spouses
who did not live together violated the patterns of time and space that characterized "normal" relationships. This challenged the taken-for-granted reality of marriage, leading members of these couples to experience "a kind of unhinging, as if
they literally felt detached from a meaning-giving unit."[18]

"Family trouble" is more complicated than a simple one-to-one relationship
between the disruption of social order and the disruption of selves, however. As
demonstrated in my examination of how parents' came to view children's behaviors and conditions as "problematic," what constitutes "family trouble" depends
upon people's collective interpretations of the situation. In fact, none of the circumstances or events discussed here are automatically troublesome. Some parents do not construct their children's poor school performances as indicative
of serious problems,[19] and some people experience relief following separation,
divorce, or the death of a family member.[20] Illness is not always disruptive and
can serve to bolster family-related identities, rather than challenge them.[21] Goffman even imagined a scenario where people accept a manic family member's
redefinitions of reality, thereby evading the family trouble stemming from mental illness.[22] In sum, there is nothing inevitable about a "problem's" construction,
and the concept of "family trouble" illuminates only those circumstances that
social actors themselves identify and experience as "problematic."[23]

Once defined as "problematic," a family's situation can be more or less troublesome, depending on the relative success of remedial efforts. In this study,
children's problems were particularly troublesome because they were so difficult to "fix." Much of the disruption stemming from undesirable conditions and
behaviors might have been curtailed had treatment programs and pharmaceutical interventions rendered children's conditions or behaviors "unproblematic"
from parents' perspectives. Just as illnesses are sometimes "cured" and couples
that entertain divorce sometimes reconcile, there are, presumably, many "problems" that have the *potential* to generate serious family trouble but are truncated
instead by people's remedial efforts.

Even when a problematic situation involves the disruption of family-related
routines and relationships, it may not have much of an impact on one's self.
Cognitive and emotional upheaval depends, in part, on the degree to which
people's self-stories are anchored to particular social patterns. As I illustrate in

previous chapters, women's greater investment in solving children's problems—and in caring for children more generally—made them more susceptible to the dynamics of family trouble featured in this text. Their sadness, guilt, and anxiety reflected narratives that were premised on the expectation of raising "healthy," "normal" children. When people's selves are less dependent on disrupted patterns, suffering is somewhat diminished. For example, uncoupling is easier for couples in long-distance relationships because each partner maintains a separate identity prior to parting ways.[24]

Because family trouble emerges in social interaction, can be curtailed by remedial efforts, and depends on people's commitments, the events and circumstances that might be analyzed within this conceptual framework are diverse. "Family trouble" is necessarily a "sensitizing concept," directing our attention to certain empirical possibilities without offering prescriptions for what we will find.[25] The degree to which a particular case of family trouble involves the features that characterized parents' troubles—the upsetting of routines, relationships, expectations, and biographical narratives—is an empirical question. Nonetheless, these patterns are basic elements of taken-for-granted reality. Since people's embeddedness in social life relies on the relative stability of these microsocial structures, it is reasonable to expect that at least some of these elements are implicated in every case of family trouble.

As parents' experiences illustrate, family trouble can pick up momentum and spill over into other areas of life, such as paid work. Because families are open systems that are embedded in and connected to other institutions, trouble can flow in and out of the family, to and from multiple directions. Employment trouble can lead to family trouble, for example,[26] and large-scale disasters usually give way to troubles of every sort.[27] In this respect, "trouble" as I have deployed it in this book has applications beyond the study of family life. The concept of "biographical disruption," conceived here as one feature of family trouble, also has broad applicability. That parents' stories are characterized by the same themes that underpin narratives of serious illness suggests that patterns of personal upheaval in late-modern life, even when they stem from different kinds of "problems," are more similar than we currently treat them. Future work might engage in a close comparison of seemingly disparate troubles seen to reside in bodies, minds, relationships, and communities.

Such an approach would need to take account of how trouble may be a feature of late-modernity itself. Parents' anxieties about children and childrearing—and the risk culture that encouraged mothers to look for potential "problems"—are in many ways a microcosm of life in the late-modern West. The constant appraisal and reappraisal of bodies, selves, and relationships are endemic to our era; we are constantly asking ourselves if everything is "okay."[28] Science contributes to this chronic reflexivity. The 20th and 21st centuries saw an explosion of prescriptive literature that identifies putative risks and advises readers on how to manage them. However, expert advice of the kind found in parenting manuals is trendy, changing from decade to decade and offering contradictory recommendations.[29] Indeed, in late-modern society, science itself is an object of endless questioning, its claims largely provisional. In this context, disruption and reorganization become the norm, as medical sociologist Simon J. Williams explains:

> Confronted with a pluralisation of life-style options and choices about everything from the food we eat to the clothes we wear, the occupations we pursue to the sexual identities we adopt, the management of our bodies and emotional selves becomes a continual process of biographical revisions and reversals, successes and failures. . . . Biographical revision, if not disruption, from this viewpoint, becomes a perennial theme in conditions of late modernity: one in which few, if any of us, are wholly immune.[30]

The benefit of "trouble" as a conceptual framework is that it offers a distinctly sociological way of talking about phenomena that are often assumed to be psychological in nature. Many of the parents in this study experienced what psychologists identify as depression and anxiety. By demonstrating how parents' cognitive and emotional turmoil were features of family trouble, this analysis places their feelings of sorrow, worry, and otherness firmly within the social realm. We need such a language. Psychiatric classifications fail to distinguish between "normal sadness" and "depressive disorder."[31] The former is a context-specific sadness that occurs in response to negative life events and can be quite intense, sharing many of the symptoms of depressive disorder. The latter is a relatively rare, long-lasting, and recurring condition characterized by reactions that are disproportionate to actual events.[32] Rather than providing an alternative framework for understanding depression, sociologists have instead adopted a psychiatric-like approach that decontextualizes sadness and "classifies a broad range of negative emotional reactions as disorders."[33] This is not a new complaint. Sociologists have all but ceded topics such as deviance to psychologists, psychiatrists, and criminologists.[34] It is not for a lack of conceptual tools that we have failed to advance sociological discourse on human suffering. As demonstrated in this book, the marriage of the concept of "personal trouble" with a structural symbolic interactionist tradition provides a fruitful avenue for exploring the social sources of personal distress.

There is much to be gained from using the concept of "trouble" to analyze upheaval in personal life. Contrary to the psychiatric point of view, which tends to pathologize negative emotions, this analysis suggests that trouble stems from an existential dilemma that is part of the human condition. As I have aimed to highlight in this book, "normalcy" is best conceptualized as an ideological (rather than empirical) category brought into sharp focus by the violation of shared expectations. The specific contours of parents' troubles may be unique, but the suffering that stems from negatively perceived difference and marginalization is a common, possibly even universal, human experience. Even so, trouble is not an altogether negative phenomenon. For some parents, it was a catalyst for positive change that deepened their understandings of themselves and the people around them. What is the role of trouble in everyday life? When does it diminish us, and when does it make us who we are? If trouble is part of what it means to be human, how can we develop a discourse that recognizes its inevitability while honoring the suffering it engenders? By continuing to explore the relationship between the disruption of social order and the disruption of selves, sociologists have an important role to play in shaping academic and public discourses on problems in personal life, intrapersonal turmoil, and human suffering.

APPENDIX A
Methods

Journalist Andrew Solomon's recent book *Far From the Tree: Parents, Children, and the Search for Identity* explores the lives of parents whose children have "horizontal identities," or identities that are strongly discordant with how parents see themselves.[1] Like this book, Solomon's work features parents whose children possess a wide array of potentially stigmatizing attributes, ranging from dwarfism to criminal pasts. Though our topic is shared, the trajectory of Solomon's book is somewhat different from this one. While I have focused largely on disruption, loss, and disconnection, Solomon's narrative is one of love, redemption, and hope. As I have noted, most published accounts of hardship foreground a "quest narrative," highlighting not chaos and darkness but what is to be *gained* from the experience.[2] Such narratives can be deeply restorative, granting the teller with agency and a sense of purpose.[3] Nonetheless, my analysis focuses particularly closely on how parents suffered.

This focus was primarily the result of early methodological choices that invited particular kinds of narrative. Part of my initial interest in this topic stemmed from a small study I had done of a public gifted program. Responding to a group of parents who had argued that giftedness is a "special need," the school district I was studying had placed nearly one-quarter of third-grade students into separate, gifted education classrooms. When I interviewed twenty of the parents who had advocated for the program's expansion, I learned that many of them had been motivated by what they saw as their children's social and academic problems. Giftedness, it seemed, was a way that some middle-class parents made sense of (what they saw as) their children's failure to perform well in ordinary classrooms. Annette Lareau's *Unequal Childhoods*[4] was released just as I was making this brief foray into the politics of special education, and, as I thought about middle-class parents' concerted efforts to raise "well-rounded," "successful" children, I became interested in what happens to middle-class parents, in this age of anxious and intensive parenting, who view their children as having "problems."

Using what is referred to as purposeful or judgmental sampling,[5] I accessed venues that I thought were most likely to yield parents who defined children's conditions or behaviors in this way. When recruiting people for the study, I explained that I was seeking to interview mothers and fathers whose children have "significant problems." There are, no doubt, parents whose children have the same conditions or behaviors as those described in this book but who do not use the interpretive framework of "problems" to describe those conditions or behaviors. Parents who consider conditions or behaviors to be "normal," "temporary," or "insignificant"—or who interpret them in terms of "difference" rather than "deviance" or "disability"—were unlikely to volunteer for a study focused on parenting children with "significant problems." What this means, though, is that the narratives featured in this book are not representative of parents whose children are different from what we imagine to be "normal." Rather, my focus is on the experiences of parents who consider their children's conditions or behaviors to be significantly "problematic." Those parents, it is reasonable to expect, are more likely to speak of disruption than mothers and fathers who make sense of the same conditions and behaviors in other ways.

I began by contacting the following four support groups: Al-Anon, a branch of Alcoholics Anonymous designed for the family members and friends of alcoholics and drug addicts; The Parent Share, a regional non-profit organization that offers support services for parents whose children have special needs; Children and Adults with Attention Deficit Disorder, or CHADD, a national organization that does support and advocacy work on behalf of children and adults with ADD/ADHD; and The Special Needs Alliance, a local support group for parents whose children have special needs. The facilitators of these groups allowed me to attend one of their meetings, briefly describe the research project, and invite their members to participate. I recruited twenty-four participants in this manner.

I recruited the remaining thirty-one participants through sources other than support or advocacy groups. A small private school for children with developmental and learning disabilities distributed information about my study to the parents of their registered students, and five of these parents volunteered for an interview. I interviewed another ten participants whose contact information I received from friends, colleagues, or other participants. And finally, I contacted three participants who were quoted in a newspaper article about therapeutic boarding schools. I was referred to the remaining thirteen participants—mostly fathers—by their current or ex-spouses.

In the end I interviewed fifty-five parents from thirty-six different families. This group included sixteen married couples, one separated couple, two divorced couples, and seventeen individuals who did not participate with a partner.[6] Categorizing children's problems is a surprisingly complicated task because some "maladies" had not been formally labeled or diagnosed, many children had more than one "problem," different conditions often shared the same "symptoms," and I almost never had the opportunity to observe children directly. Table 1 is a loose and imperfect categorization of children's primary or most pressing problems, but it effectively conveys the variation in my sample.

Table 1   Summary of Children's Primary Problems

Types of Problem	N
Attention deficit/hyperactivity disorder and learning disabilities (including dyslexia, auditory processing disorder, and non-specific learning disabilities)	5
Developmental disabilities (including conditions on the autism spectrum; delays related to brain injuries, seizure disorders, cerebral palsy, Fragile X syndrome, and fetal alcohol syndrome; and non-specific delays)	16
Mental health problems (including depression, attempted suicide, attachment disorder, trichotillomania, bipolar disorder, and non-specific behavioral problems such as aggression)	10
Substance abuse or addiction	12
Medical condition (without developmental disabilities)	1
Total	44*

* Some participating families had more than one child with problems. This is why the total number of children in the sample is forty-four, even though there are only thirty-six participating families.

In addition to having a range of conditions and behaviors, children varied in terms of age, gender, and kinship status. At the time of the interviews, children's ages ranged from five to forty-four years old, although approximately two-thirds were under the age of eighteen and living with their parents at the time of the interview.[7] Although there was a disproportionate number of boys (twenty-five sons, as opposed to nineteen daughters), girls were represented in each problem category. Seven children were adopted. See Appendix B for a complete reference of each child's age, gender, kinship status, and problem summary.

Table 2   Parents' Incomes

Annual Household Income	N
$30,000–$50,000	7
$51,000–$70,000	8
$71,000–$90,000	6
$91,000–$110,000	10
$111,000–250,000	6
Total	37*

* Divorced couples' incomes are reported separately. One couple preferred not to report their household income.

With few exceptions, the parents I interviewed were middle class as defined by income, education level, and home ownership status. Their annual household incomes average at $93,000, ranging from $30,000 to $250,000, as illustrated in Table 2. All but three families made at least $50,000 per year, and all but five owned their own homes. As illustrated in Table 3, most participants had post-secondary degrees.

Table 3   Educational Level of Parents

Degree	N (Fathers)	N (Mothers)
High School Diploma	2	8
Associate's Degree	2	3
Bachelor's Degree	9	12
Post-Graduate Degree	8	11
Total	21	34

I asked parents to choose the location of our conversations, and I interviewed most in their homes, cafes and restaurants, and places of employment. Six married couples preferred to be interviewed together, but I talked with the remaining mothers and fathers separately. Following an inductive approach, I structured the interviews very loosely, thinking of them as "guided conversations" rather than a static set of questions and responses.[8] I opened each conversation by asking parents to describe their children and to tell me the story of their problems. I encouraged participants at the outset to emphasize what had been the most salient aspects of their experiences, while also prompting them to discuss how their children came to be identified as having problems, the perceived source(s) of those problems, and their efforts to help their children. Our meetings ranged in length from forty-five minutes to three hours.

Having come to this study interested in parents' role in the problematization of childhood and the politics of educational inequality, it was only after I started doing interviews that I came to realize just how disruptive children's problems had been. I was surprised initially that even comparatively mild "problems," such as learning disabilities, challenged parents' taken-for-granted realities, interrupted the flow of their daily activities, played havoc with their close personal relationships, and brought them to tears. When I realized the deep and wide-ranging impacts of children's problems on parents' lives, I shifted the focus of my research and started to ask parents more specifically about how children's problems had changed their notions of self, worldviews, marriages, friendships, and social lives. I learned, ultimately, that the topic of parents' troubles was not separate from my initial interests. The longer I listened to parents' stories, the more I realized that their attempts to label and treat children's problems were inextricably bound to their own suffering. In many ways, to trace the career of children's problems—from onset and recognition, to naming and treatment—is to trace the career of parents' troubles. As I have argued in this book, parents' actions stemmed not only from a desire to help their children, but also from their efforts to manage uncertainty and stigma, remain within the boundaries of "normal" middle-class life, cope with guilt and grief, and restructure their identities in ways that re-secured them to social life.

APPENDIX B

Participants

Parent(s) Names	Kinship Status	Child's Age	Child's Gender	Primary Problem(s)
Megan & Craig	Biological parents	16	Daughter	Depression, attempted suicide
Rachel & Joel	Biological parents	13	Daughter	Attempted suicide, attempted to run away
Susan	Biological parent	16	Daughter	Trichotillomania, poor academic performance
Joan & Sergio	Biological parents	15	Son	Mental illness (no specific diagnosis)
Cynthia & Russell	Biological parents	18	Daughter	Depression
Carol	Biological parent	13	Son	Asperger's syndrome
Marie & Steve	Biological parents	17	Daughter	Cocaine addiction
Claire	Biological parent	9	Son	Autism
Deborah	Biological parent	23	Son	Alcoholism
Peg	Biological parent	16	Son	Attention deficit disorder, learning disabilities
Grace & Sam	Adoptive parents	17	Daughter	Attention deficit disorder, depression, poor academic performance
Sarah & Matt	Biological / adoptive parents	13	Son	Severe brain injury, developmental disabilities
	Adoptive / biological parents	17	Son	Drug abuse
Mary & Phil	Biological parents	17	Son	Drug abuse, selling drugs

Participants (*continued*)

Cindy	Biological parent	44	Son	Alcoholism, drug addiction
	Biological parent	40	Son	Alcoholism, drug addiction
	Stepparent	38	Son	Alcoholism, drug addiction
	Stepparent	27	Daughter	Alcoholism, drug addiction
	Stepparent	24	Daughter	Alcoholism, drug addiction
Valerie & Keith	Biological parents	11	Daughter	Autism
Jessica & Peter	Biological parents	6	Son	Mental illness (no specific diagnosis)
Jen & Carl	Adoptive parents	13	Daughter	Attachment disorder
	Adoptive parents	8	Daughter	Fetal alcohol syndrome
Kathy	Biological parent	6	Son	Cerebral palsy, developmental disabilities
Lauren	Adoptive parent	10	Daughter	Developmental disability
	Adoptive parent	10	Daughter	Developmental disability
Anna	Biological parent	21	Daughter	Developmental disability
Lisa	Biological parent	9	Son	Hyperinsulinism, developmental disabilities
	Biological parent	5	Daughter	Hyperinsulinism[*]
Judy & Tom	Biological parents	25	Son	Attention deficit disorder
Andrea	Biological parent	19	Daughter	Drug addiction, aggression

Paula & Mike	Biological parents	8	Son	Attention deficit disorder
Seth & Rhonda	Biological parents	19	Daughter	Drug addiction, ran away for an extended period
Diane	Biological parent	21	Daughter	Drug addiction, unplanned pregnancy, poor academic performance
Jason & Monica	Biological parents	6	Son	Autism
Eve & Tim	Biological parents	17	Son	Fragile X syndrome, developmental disabilities
Martha & Henry	Biological parents	13	Daughter	Dyslexia
Sandra & Doug	Adoptive parents	13	Son	Aggression, behavioral problems (no specific diagnosis)
Daniel	Biological parent	18	Son	Attention deficit disorder, auditory processing disorder, learning disabilities
Patty	Biological parent	13	Son	Autism
Jody	Biological parent	19	Son	Cerebral palsy, developmental disabilities
Olivia & Jerry	Adoptive parents	10	Son	Brain injury, behavioral problems (no specific diagnosis), learning disabilities
Amanda	Biological parent	15	Son	Bipolar disorder
Bill	Biological parent	16	Son	Seizure disorder (nonspecific), developmental disabilities

* In the case of Lisa's daughter, hyperinsulinism was a strictly physical condition that did not impact her development.

NOTES

CHAPTER 1 PARENTS IN TROUBLE

1. In order to protect participants' confidentiality, I use pseudonyms for all parents and their children.

2. David R. Maines, *The Faultline of Consciousness: A View of Interactionism in Sociology* (New York: Aldine De Gruyter, 2001).

3. David A. Snow and Leon Anderson, *Down on Their Luck: A Study of Homeless Street People* (Berkeley, CA: University of California Press, 1993), 288.

4. Peter L. Berger, *Invitation to Sociology: A Humanistic Perspective* (Garden City: Doubleday, 1963), 148.

5. Ibid., 148–149.

6. Ibid., 138.

7. Harold Garfinkel, "Studies of the Routine Grounds of Everyday Activities," *Social Problems* 11 (1964): 225–250.

8. Edward Gross and Gregory P. Stone, "Embarrassment and the Analysis of Role Requirements," *American Journal of Sociology* 70 (1964): 1–15.

9. C. Wright Mills, *The Sociological Imagination* (New York: Oxford University Press, 1959).

10. Robert M. Emerson and Sheldon L. Messinger, "The Micro-Politics of Trouble." *Social Problems* 25 (1977): 121–135; Robert M. Emerson, "Responding to Roommate Troubles: Reconsidering Informal Dyadic Control," *Law & Society Review* 42 (2008): 483–512; Robert M. Emerson, "Ethnography, Interaction and Ordinary Trouble," *Ethnography* 10 (2009): 535–548; Robert M. Emerson, "From Normal Conflict to Normative Deviance: The Micro-Politics of Trouble in Close Relationships," *Journal of Contemporary Ethnography* 40 (2011): 3–38.

11. Gail Jefferson, "On 'Trouble-Premonitory' Response to Inquiry," *Sociological Inquiry* 50 (1980): 153–185.

12. Judith Butler, *Gender Trouble: Feminism and the Subversion of Identity* (New York: Routledge, 1990).

13. Jefferson, "On 'Trouble-Premonitory' Response to Inquiry," 153.

14. Emerson, "From Normal Conflict to Normative Deviance," 7.

15. Butler, *Gender Trouble*.

16. David Cheal, "Unity and Difference in Postmodern Families," *Journal of Family Issues* 14 (1993): 5–19; Andrew J. Cherlin, "The Deinstitutionalization of American Marriage," *Journal of Marriage and Family* 66 (2004): 848–861; Stephanie Coontz, *Marriage, A History: From Obedience to Intimacy, or How Love Conquered Marriage* (Berkeley, CA: University of California Press, 2005).

17. Sheldon Stryker and Peter J. Burke, "The Past, Present, and Future of Identity Theory," *Social Psychology Quarterly*, 63 (2000): 284–297.

18. Andrew J. Weigert and Ross Hastings, "Identity Loss, Family, and Social Change," *American Journal of Sociology* 82 (1977): 1171–1185.

19. Erving Goffman, "The Insanity of Place," in *Relations in Public: Micro Studies of Public Order* (New York: Basic Books, 1971), 335–390.

20. Ibid., 367.

21. Lyn Craig and Killian Mullan, "Parenthood, Gender and Work–Family Time in the United States, Australia, Italy, France, and Denmark," *Journal of Marriage and Family* 72 (2010): 1344–1361.

22. Amy Claxton and Maureen Perry-Jenkins, "No Fun Anymore: Leisure and Marital Quality Across the Transition to Parenthood," *Journal of Marriage and Family* 70 (2008): 28–43.

23. Sarah A. Burgard and Jennifer A. Ailshire, "Gender and Time for Sleep among U.S. Adults," *American Sociological Review* 78 (2012): 51–69. Mothers are disproportionately affected by the temporal demands of caregiving, but today's fathers spend more time performing routine childcare than ever before, see Suzanne M. Bianchi, John P. Robinson, and Melissa A. Milkie, *Changing Rhythms of American Family Life* (New York: Russell Sage Foundation, 2006).

24. Knud Knudsen and Kari Wærness, "National Context and Spouses' Housework in 34 Countries," *European Sociological Review* 24 (2008): 97–113.

25. Kelly K. Bost, Martha J. Cox, and Chris Payne, "Structural and Supportive Changes in Couples' Family and Friendship Networks Across the Transition to Parenthood," *Journal of Marriage and Family* 64 (2002): 517–531.

26. See Jennifer Lois, *Home Is Where the School Is: The Logic of Homeschooling and the Emotional Labor of Mothering* (New York: New York University Press, 2012), Part I.

27. Robin W. Simon, "The Joys of Parenthood, Reconsidered," *Contexts* 7 (2008): 40–45.

28. Everett C. Hughes, "Dilemmas and Contradictions of Status" *American Journal of Sociology* 50 (1945): 357.

29. Alice Kessler-Harris, *Out to Work: A History of Wage-Earning Women in the United States* (New York: Oxford University Press, 2003).

30. Bianchi, Robinson, and Milkie, *Changing Rhythms of American Family Life*; Linda J. Waite and Mark Nielsen, "The Rise of the Dual-Worker Family: 1963–1997," in *Working Families: The Transformation of the American Home* ed. Rosanna Hertz and Nancy L. Marshall (Berkeley, CA: University of California Press, 2001), 23–41.

31. Suzanne M. Bianchi, "Family Change and Time Allocation in American Families," *The Annals of The American Academy of Political and Social Science* 638 (2011): 21–44.

32. Bianchi, Robinson, and Milkie, *Changing Rhythms of American Family Life*.

33. Ibid.

34. Ibid.

35. Arland Thornton and Linda Young-DeMarco, "Four Decades of Trends in Attitudes toward Family Issues in the United States: The 1960s through the 1990s," *Journal of Marriage and the Family* 63 (2001): 1009–1037; Tanya Koropeckyj-Cox and Gretchen Pendell, "Attitudes About Childlessness in the United States: Correlates of Positive, Neutral, and Negative Responses," *Journal of Family Issues* 28 (2007): 1054–1082.

36. Philippe Ariès, *Centuries of Childhood* (London: Jonathan Cape Ltd., 1962); Viviana A. Zelizer, *Pricing the Priceless Child: The Changing Social Value of Children* (Princeton, NJ: Princeton University Press, 1985); Peter Stearns, *Anxious Parents: A History of Modern Childrearing in America* (New York: New York University Press, 2003).

37. Zelizer, *Pricing the Priceless Child: The Changing Social Value of Children*.

38. Tamara K. Hareven, *Families, History, and Social Change: Life course & Cross Cultural Perspectives* (Boulder, CO: Westview Press, 2000).

39. John R. Gillis, *A World of Their Own Making* (Cambridge, MA: Harvard University Press, 1996).

40. Allison Pugh, *Longing and Belonging: Parents, Children, and Consumer Culture* (Berkeley, CA: University of California Press, 2009), 20.

41. George Herbert Mead, *Mind, Self, and Society* (Chicago: University of Chicago Press, 1934).

42. Anselm Strauss, *Mirrors and Masks* (Glencoe: Free Press, 1959), 91.

43. Strauss, *Mirrors and Masks*; Agnes Hankiss, "Ontologies of the Self: On the Mythological Rearranging of One's Life History," in *Biography and Society: The Life History Approach in the Social Sciences*, ed. Daniel Bertaux (Los Angeles, CA: Sage Publications, 1981), 203–209; Kenneth J. Gergen and Mary M. Gergen, "Narratives of the Self" in *Studies in Social Identity*, ed. Theodore R. Sarbin and Karl E. Scheibe (New York: Praeger, 1983), 254–273; Gaylene Becker, *Disrupted Lives: How People Create Meaning in a Chaotic World* (Berkeley, CA: University of California Press, 1997).

44. Gergen and Gergen, "Narratives of the Self."

45. Becker, *Disrupted Lives*, 5.

46. See Eviatar Zerubavel, *Time Maps: Collective Memory and the Social Shape of the Past* (Chicago: University of Chicago Press, 2003), 14–15.

47. Strauss, *Mirrors and Masks*, 132–147.

48. Ibid., 93.

49. Michael Bury, "Chronic Illness as Biographical Disruption," *Sociology of Health and Illness* 4 (1982): 167–182.

50. Arthur W. Frank, *The Wounded Storyteller: Body, Illness, and Ethics* (Chicago: University of Chicago Press, 1995).

51. See also Bridget Young, Mary Dixon-Woods, Michelle Findlay, and David Heney, "Parenting in a Crisis: Conceptualising Mothers of Children with Cancer," *Social Science & Medicine* 55 (2002): 1835–1847.

52. Gergen and Gergen, "Narratives of the Self."

53. See Joan B. Wolf, *Is Breast Best?: Taking on the Breastfeeding Experts and the New High Stakes of Motherhood* (New York: New York University Press, 2011).

54. Sharon Hays, *Cultural Contradictions of Motherhood* (New Haven, CT: Yale University Press, 1996).

55. Peter Conrad and Joseph Schneider, *Deviance and Medicalization, From Badness to Sickness* (St. Louis, NO: Mosby Publishing Company, 1980); Peter Conrad, *The Medicalization of Society: On the Transformation of Human Conditions into Treatable Disorders* (Baltimore: Johns Hopkins University Press, 2007).

56. Lennard J. Davis, *Enforcing Normalcy: Disability, Deafness, and the Body* (London: Verso, 1995), 23–49; for a discussion of norms and ideals pertaining to families, see Gillis, *A World of Their Own Making*, 3–40.

57. Davis, *Enforcing Normalcy*, 23–49.

58. Dorothy E. Smith, "The Standard North American Family: SNAF as an Ideological Code," *Journal of Family Issues* 14 (1993), 50–65; James A. Holstein and Jaber F. Gubrium, "Deprivatization and the Construction of Domestic Life," *Journal of Marriage and The Family* 57 (1995), 894–908; Judith Stacey, "The Right Family Values," in *Families in the U.S.: Kinship and Domestic Policies*, ed. Karen Hansen and Anita I. Garey (Philadelphia: Temple University Press, 1998), 859–880.

59. Davis, *Enforcing Normalcy*, 23–49.

60. See, for example, John Swain, Sally French, Colin Barnes, and Carol Thomas, eds., *Disabling Barriers, Enabling Environments* (London: Sage, 2004).

61. Michael Oliver, *The Politics of Disablement: A Sociological Approach* (London: Palgrave Macmillan, 1990).

62. For a thorough discussion see Simon J. Williams, "Chronic Illness as Biographical Disruption or Biographical Disruption as Chronic Illness? Reflections on a Core Concept," *Sociology of Health and Illness* 22 (2000): 40–67.

63. W. I. Thomas and Dorothy Swaine Thomas, *The Child in America: Behavior Problems and Programs* (New York: Knopf, 1928), 572.

64. Erving Goffman, *Stigma: Notes on the Management of Spoiled Identity* (New York: Aronson, 1963), 127.

65. Becker, *Disrupted Lives*.

66. Ibid., 5–7.

67. Eviatar Zerubavel, "Generally Speaking: The Logic and Mechanics of Social Pattern Analysis," *Sociological Forum* 22 (2007): 141.

68. Ibid., 134–136.

69. For a more thorough discussion, see Zerubavel, "Generally Speaking."

70. Goffman, *Stigma*.

71. Eviatar Zerubavel, *Hidden Rhythms: Schedules and Calendars in Social Life* (Chicago: University of Chicago Press, 1981).

72. Diane Vaughan, *Uncoupling*, (New York: Oxford University Press, 1986).

73. Helen Rose Fuchs Ebaugh, *Becoming an Ex: The Process of Role Exit* (Chicago: University of Chicago Press, 1988).

74. For a discussion of "sensitizing concepts," see Herbert Blumer, *Symbolic Interaction: Perspective and Method* (Berkeley, CA: University of California Press, 1969), 149–152.

75. Bianchi, Robinson, and Milkie, *Changing Rhythms of American Family Life*.

76. Ibid.

77. Annette Lareau, *Unequal Childhoods: Class, Race and Family Life* (Berkeley, CA: University of California Press, 2003).

78. Jane R. Mercer, "Social System Perspective and Clinical Perspective: Frames of Reference for Understanding Career Patterns of Persons Labeled as Mental Retarded," *Social Problems* 13 (1965): 18–34; Beth Harry, "Making Sense of Disability: Low-Income, Puerto Rican Parents' Theories of the Problem," *Exceptional Children* 59 (1992): 27–40.

CHAPTER 2 CONSTRUCTING TROUBLE, LOSING CERTAINTY

1. Robert M. Emerson and Sheldon L. Messinger, "The Micro-Politics of Trouble." *Social Problems* 25 (1977): 121–135.

2. See Joan B. Wolf, *Is Breast Best?: Taking on the Breastfeeding Experts and the New High Stakes of Motherhood* (New York: New York University Press, 2011).

3. Sharon Hays, *Cultural Contradictions of Motherhood* (New Haven, CT: Yale University Press, 1996).

4. Peter Conrad and Joseph Schneider, *Deviance and Medicalization, From Badness to Sickness* (St. Louis, MO: Mosby Publishing Company, 1980); Adam Rafalovich, "Attention Deficit-Hyperactivity Disorder as the Medicalization of Childhood: Challenges from and for Sociology," *Sociology Compass* 7 (2013): 343–354.

5. Peter Stearns, *Anxious Parents: A History of Modern Childrearing in America* (New York: New York University Press, 2003).

6. See Wolf, *Is Breast Best?*

7. Stearns, *Anxious Parents*.

8. See also Ilina Singh, "Boys Will Be Boys: Fathers' Perspectives on ADHD Symptoms, Diagnosis and Drug Treatment," *Harvard Review of Psychiatry* 11 (2003): 308–316.

9. Emerson and Messinger, "The Micro-Politics of Trouble," 121.

10. Charles Rosenberg and Janet Golden, *Framing Disease: Studies in Cultural History* (New Brunswick, NJ: Rutgers University Press, 1992), xxiv.

11. Hays, *Cultural Contradictions of Motherhood*, x.

12. See, for example, Molly Ladd-Taylor and Lauri Umansky, eds., *"Bad" Mothers: The Politics of Blame in Twentieth Century America* (New York: New York University Press, 1998).

13. Wolf, *Is Breast Best?*

14. See also Singh, "Boys Will Be Boys."

15. Kathy Charmaz, *Good Days, Bad Days* (New Brunswick, NJ: Rutgers University Press, 1991).

16. Rafalovich, "Attention Deficit-Hyperactivity Disorder as the Medicalization of Childhood."

17. Emerson and Messinger, "The Micro-Politics of Trouble."

18. Christopher Adamson, "Existential and Clinical Uncertainty in The Medical Encounter: An Idiographic Account of an Illness Trajectory Defined by Inflammatory Bowel Disease and Avascular Necrosis," *Sociology Of Health & Illness* 19 (1997): 133–159; Renee C. Fox, "Medical Uncertainty Revisited," in *The Handbook of Social Studies in Health and Medicine*, eds. Gary L. Albrecht, Ray Fitzpatrick, and Susan C. Scrimshaw (London: Sage, 2000), 409–425; Andrea Stockl, "Complex Syndromes, Ambivalent Diagnosis, and Existential Uncertainty: The Case of Systemic Lupus Erythematosus (SLE)," *Social Science & Medicine* 65 (2007): 1549–1559.

19. David A. Karp, *Speaking of Sadness: Depression, Disconnection, and the Meanings of Illness* (New York: Oxford University Press, 1997); Renee L. Beard and Patrick J. Fox, "Resisting Social Disenfranchisement: Negotiating Collective Identities and Everyday Life with Memory Loss," *Social Science & Medicine* 66 (2008): 1509–1520.

20. Fox, "Medical Uncertainty Revisited."

21. Adamson, "Existential and Clinical Uncertainty in The Medical Encounter"; Stockl, "Complex Syndromes, Ambivalent Diagnosis, and Existential Uncertainty."

22. Robert Byrd, Allyson C. Sage, and Janet Keyzer, "Report to the Legislature on the Principal Findings of the Epidemiology of Autism in California: A Comprehensive Pilot Study," MIND Institute, 2002.

23. Pamela Kidder-Ashley, James R. Deni, and Jessica B. Anderton, "Learning Disabilities Eligibility in the 1990s: Analysis of State Practices," *Education* 121 (2000): 65–73.

24. Maia Szalavitz, *Help at Any Cost: How the Troubled-Teen Industry Cons Parents and Hurts Kids* (London: Penguin Books, 2006).

25. See Erving Goffman, "The Insanity of Place," in *Relations in Public: Micro Studies of Public Order* (New York: Basic Books, 1971), 335–390.

CHAPTER 3 ELUSIVE REMEDIES AND DISRUPTED ROUTINES

1. "Coalition for Autism Intervention" is a pseudonym.

2. Arthur W. Frank, *The Wounded Storyteller: Body, Illness, and Ethics* (Chicago: University of Chicago Press, 1995), 75–96.

3. Annette Lareau, *Unequal Childhoods: Class, Race and Family Life* (Berkeley, CA: University of California Press, 2003).

4. Ellen Brantlinger, *Dividing Classes: How the Middle Class Negotiates and Rationalizes School Advantage* (New York: Routledge, 2003).

5. Linda Blum, "Mother-Blame in the Prozac Nation: Raising Kids with Invisible Disabilities," *Gender & Society* 21 (2007): 202–226.

6. Ibid., 222.

7. Jacquelyn Litt, "Women's Carework in Low-Income Households: The Special Case of Children with Attention Deficit Hyperactivity Disorder," *Gender & Society* 18 (2004): 625–644.

8. Peter Conrad, "The Shifting Engines of Medicalization," *Journal of Health and Social Behavior* 46 (2005): 3–14.

9. Ibid., 8–9.

10. Wade F. Horn and Douglas Tynan, "Revamping Special Education," *Public Interest* 114 (2001): 36–53.

11. Ibid.

12. Ibid.

13. Laudan Aron and Pamela Loprest, "Disability and the Education System," *Future of Children* 22 (2012): 97–122.

14. Horn and Tynan, "Revamping Special Education"; Gerald Coles, *The Learning Mystique* (New York: Pantheon Books, 1987).

15. Aron and Loprest, "Disability and the Education System."

16. Blum, "Mother-Blame in the Prozac Nation."

17. Horn and Tynan, "Revamping Special Education"; Aron and Loprest, "Disability and the Education System," 110.

18. Although the federal government can cover up to 40 percent of special education costs, their funding has never come close to meeting this cap. In 1999–2000, they covered only 9 percent of special education costs, nationwide. States covered 45 percent, and the remaining 46 percent was covered by local school districts. See Aron and Loprest, "Disability and the Education System," 110.

19. See also Blum, "Mother-Blame in the Prozac Nation."

20. Claudia Malacrida, "Medicalization, Ambivalence, and Social Control: Mothers' Descriptions of Educators and ADD/ADHD," *Health: An Interdisciplinary Journal for the Social Study of Health, Illness and Medicine* 8 (2004): 61–80.

21. See Blum, "Mother-Blame in the Prozac Nation"; Litt, "Women's Carework in Low-Income Households."

22. Also see Malacrida, "Medicalization, Ambivalence, and Social Control."

23. Shari L. Thurer, *The Myths of Motherhood: How Culture Reinvents the Good Mother* (Boston: Houghton Mifflin Company, 1994).

24. See, for example, Jennifer Lois, *Home Is Where the School Is: The Logic of Homeschooling and the Emotional Labor of Mothering* (New York: New York University Press, 2012).

25. Eviatar Zerubavel, *Hidden Rhythms: Schedules and Calendars in Social Life* (Chicago: University of Chicago Press, 1981).

26. Gaylene Becker, *Disrupted Lives: How People Create Meaning in a Chaotic World* (Berkeley, CA: University of California Press, 1997), 4.

CHAPTER 4 STIGMA AND DISRUPTED RELATIONSHIPS

1. Erving Goffman, *Stigma: Notes on the Management of Spoiled Identity* (New York: Aronson, 1963), 30.

2. A portion of this chapter appeared as "Stigma in an Era of Medicalisation and Anxious Parenting: How Proximity and Culpability Shape Middle-Class Parents' Experiences of Disgrace," *Sociology of Health and Illness* 34 (2012): 927–942.

3. Peter L. Berger and Hansfried Kellner, "Marriage and the Construction of Reality: A Contribution to the Microsociology of Knowledge," *Diogenes* 12 (1964): 1–24; Philip Blumstein, "The Production of Selves in Personal Relationships," in *The Self-Society Dynamic: Cognition,*

Emotional, and Action, ed. Judith A. Howard and Peter L. Callero (New York: Cambridge University Press, 1991), 205–322.

4. See, for example, Lyn H. Lofland, "Loss and Human Connection: An Exploration into the Nature of the Social Bond," in *Personality, Roles, and Social Behavior*, ed. William Ickes and Eric S. Knowles (New York: Springer-Verlag, 1982), 219–242; Diane Vaughan, *Uncoupling* (New York: Oxford University Press, 1986).

5. Erving Goffman, "The Insanity of Place," in *Relations in Public: Micro Studies of Public Order* (New York: Basic Books, 1971), 367.

6. Goffman, *Stigma*, 30.

7. Arnold Birenbaum, "On Managing Courtesy Stigma," *Journal of Health and Social Behavior* 11 (1970): 196–206; David Gray, "High Functioning Autistic Children and the Construction of 'Normal' Family Life," *Social Science and Medicine* 44 (1997): 1097–1106; David Gray, "'Everybody Just Freezes. Everybody is Just Embarrassed': Felt and Enacted Stigma among Parents of Children with High Functioning Autism," *Sociology of Health and Illness* 24 (2002): 734–749; Sara E. Green, "'Oh, Those Therapists will Become Your Best Friends': Maternal Satisfaction with Clinics Providing Physical, Occupational and Speech Therapy Services to Children with Disabilities," *Sociology of Health & Illness* 23 (2001): 798–828; Sara E. Green, "What Do You Mean 'What's Wrong with Her?': Stigma and the Lives of Families of Children with Disabilities," *Social Science & Medicine* 57 (2003): 1361–1374; Sara E. Green, "The Impact of Stigma on Maternal Attitudes toward Placement of Children with Disabilities in Residential Care Facilities," *Social Science & Medicine* 59 (2004): 799–812; Kristin D. Mickelson, "Perceived Stigma, Social Support, and Depression," *Personality and Social Psychology Bulletin* 27 (2001): 1046–1056; Sara E. Green et al., "Living Stigma: The Impact of Labeling, Stereotyping, Separation, Status Loss, and Discrimination in the Lives of Individuals with Disabilities and Their Families," *Sociological Inquiry* 75 (2005): 197–215; Mirka Koro-Ljungberg and Regina Bussing, "The Management of Courtesy Stigma in the Lives of Families with Teenagers with ADHD," *Journal of Family Issues* 30 (2009): 1175–2000; David Farrugia, "Exploring Stigma: Medical Knowledge and the Stigmatisation of Parents of Children Diagnosed with Autism Spectrum Disorder," *Sociology of Health & Illness* 31 (2009): 1011–1027.

8. Graham Scambler and Anthony Hopkins, "Being Epileptic: Coming to Terms with Stigma," *Sociology of Health and Illness* 8 (1986): 26–43; Gray, "'Everybody Just Freezes. Everybody is Just Embarrassed'"; Green et al., "Living Stigma."

9. Green, "What Do You Mean 'What's Wrong with Her?'"; Green, "The Impact of Stigma on Maternal Attitudes."

10. Mickelson, "Perceived Stigma, Social Support, and Depression."

11. Suzanne M. Bianchi, John P. Robinson, and Melissa A. Milkie, *Changing Rhythms of American Family Life* (New York: Russell Sage Foundation, 2006).

12. Shari L. Thurer, *The Myths of Motherhood: How Culture Reinvents the Good Mother* (Boston: Houghton Mifflin Company, 1994); Sharon Hays, *Cultural Contradictions of Motherhood* (New Haven, CT: Yale University Press, 1996); Susan Douglas and Meredith Michaels, *The Mommy Myth* (New York: Free Press, 2004).

13. Hays, *The Cultural Contradictions of Motherhood*; Annette Lareau, *Unequal Childhoods: Class, Race and Family Life* (Berkeley, CA: University of California Press, 2003).

14. Thurer, *The Myths of Motherhood*; Molly Ladd-Taylor and Lauri Umansky, eds., *"Bad" Mothers: The Politics of Blame in Twentieth Century America* (New York: New York University Press, 1998); Anita Garey and Terry Arendell, "Children, Work, and Family: Some Thoughts on 'Mother-Blame,'" in *Working Families: The Transformation of the American Home*, ed. Rosanna Hertz and Nancy Marshall (Berkeley, CA: University of California Press, 2001), 293–303.

15. Douglas and Michaels, *The Mommy Myth*, 8.

16. Goffman, *Stigma*, 4.

17. Peter Conrad and Joseph Schneider, *Deviance and Medicalization, From Badness to Sickness* (St. Louis, MO: Mosby Publishing Company, 1980); Peter Conrad, *The Medicalization of Society: On the Transformation of Human Conditions into Treatable Disorders* (Baltimore: The Johns Hopkins University Press, 2007).

18. Conrad and Schneider, *Deviance and Medicalization*; Linda Blum, "Mother-Blame in the Prozac Nation: Raising Kids with Invisible Disabilities," *Gender & Society* 21 (2007): 202–226; Jack K. Martin, Bernice A. Pescosolido, Sigrun Olafsdottir, and Jane D. McLeod, "The Construction of Fear: Americans' Preferences for Social Distance from Children and Adolescents with Mental Health Problems," *Journal of Health and Social Behavior* 48 (2007): 50–67; Patrick W. Corrigan, Amy C. Watson, and Fredrick E. Miller, "Blame, Shame, and Contamination: The Impact of Mental Illness and Drug Dependence Stigma on Family Members," *Journal of Family Psychology* 20 (2006): 239–246.

19. Janet Golden, *Message in a Bottle* (Cambridge, MA: Harvard University Press, 2005); Peter Stearns, *Anxious Parents: A History of Modern Childrearing in America* (New York: New York University Press, 2003).

20. Claudia Malacrida, *Cold Comfort: Mothers, Professionals, and Attention Deficit (Hyperactivity) Disorder* (Toronto: University of Toronto Press, 2003); Jacquelyn Litt, "Women's Carework in Low-Income Households: The Special Case of Children with Attention Deficit Hyperactivity Disorder," *Gender & Society* 18 (2004): 625–644; Ilina Singh, "Doing Their Jobs: Mothering with Ritalin in a Culture of Mother-Blame," *Social Science and Medicine* 59 (2004): 1193–1205.

21. Lynn M. Appleton, "Rethinking Medicalization: Alcoholism and Anomalies," in *Images of Issues*, ed. Joel Best (Hawthorne: Aldine de Gruyter, 1995); Carl May, "Pathology, Identity and the Social Construction of Alcohol Dependence," *Sociology* 35 (2001): 385–401.

22. David Gray, "High Functioning Autistic Children."

23. See also Farrugia, "Exploring Stigma."

24. Masako Ishii-Kuntz and Karen Seccombe, "The Impact of Children upon Social Support Networks Throughout the Life Course," *Journal of Marriage and the Family* 51 (1989): 777–790.

25. Sally K. Gallagher and Naomi Gerstel, "Connections and Constraints: The Effects of Children on Caregiving," *Journal of Marriage and the Family* 63 (2001): 265–275.

26. See, for example, Bridget Byrne, "In Search of a 'Good Mix': 'Race,' Class, Gender and Practices of Mothering," *Sociology* 40 (2006): 1001–1017.

27. Melissa A. Milkie, Suzanne M. Bianchi, Marybeth J. Mattingly, and John P. Robinson, "Gendered Division of Childrearing: Ideals, Realities, and the Relationship to Parental Well-Being," *Sex Roles* 47 (2002): 21–38.

28. Viviana A. Zelizer, *Pricing the Priceless Child: The Changing Social Value of Children* (Princeton, NJ: Princeton University Press, 1985); Peter Stearns, *Anxious Parents: A History of Modern Childrearing in America* (New York: New York University Press, 2003).

CHAPTER 5   UNMET EXPECTATIONS AND EMOTIONAL TURMOIL

1. Harold Garfinkel, "Studies of the Routine Grounds of Everyday Activities," *Social Problems* 11 (1964): 225–250.

2. Stephanie Coontz, *Marriage, A History: From Obedience to Intimacy, or How Love Conquered Marriage* (Berkeley, CA: University of California Press, 2005).

3. Kathryn Edin and Maria J. Kefalas, *Promises I Can Keep: Why Poor Women Put Motherhood Before Marriage* (Berkeley, CA: University of California Press, 2005).

4. Garfinkel, "Studies of the Routine Grounds of Everyday Activities."

5. Kathy Charmaz and Melinda Milligan, "Grief," in *Handbook of the Sociology of Emotions*, eds. Jan E. Stets and Jonathan H. Turner (New York: Springer, 2007), 516–543.

6. Annette Mahoney, Kenneth I. Pargament, Aaron Murray-Swank, and Nichole Murray-Swank, "Religion and the Sanctification of Family Relationships," *Review of Religious Research* 44 (2003): 220–236.

7. Jennifer Lois, *Home Is Where the School Is: The Logic of Homeschooling and the Emotional Labor of Mothering* (New York: New York University Press, 2012), 42.

8. Pauline Boss, "Ambiguous Loss Research, Theory, and Practice," *Journal of Marriage and Family* 66 (2004): 551–566.

9. Ibid., 553–554.

10. Candace Clarke, *Misery and Company: Sympathy in Everyday Life* (Chicago: University of Chicago Press, 1998).

11. Lois, *Home Is Where the School Is*.

12. Ibid.

13. See also Nina Hallowell et al., "Guilt, Blame, and Responsibility: Men's Understanding of Their Role in the Transmission of BRCA1/2 Mutations Within Their Family," *Sociology of Health & Illness* 28 (2006): 969–988.

14. Joan B. Wolf, *Is Breast Best?: Taking on the Breastfeeding Experts and the New High Stakes of Motherhood* (New York: New York University Press, 2011), xvi.

15. See, for example, Judith Warner, *Perfect Madness: Motherhood in the Age of Anxiety* (New York: Riverhead Books, 2005).

16. For exceptions see Ilina Singh, "Boys Will Be Boys: Fathers' Perspectives on ADHD Symptoms, Diagnosis and Drug Treatment," *Harvard Review of Psychiatry* 11 (2003): 308–316; and Fiona Shirani, Karen Henwood, and Carrie Coltart, "Meeting the Challenges of Intensive Parenting Culture: Gender, Risk, Management, and the Moral Parent," *Sociology* 46 (2012): 25–40.

17. Sheldon Stryker and Peter J. Burke, "The Past, Present, and Future of Identity Theory," *Social Psychology Quarterly* 63 (2000): 284–297.

18. Peter J. Burke and Donald C. Reitzes, "An Identity Theory Approach to Commitment," *Social Psychology Quarterly* 54 (1991): 239–251; Stryker and Burke, "The Past, Present, and Future of Identity Theory."

19. Peter J. Burke and Jan E. Stets, "Trust and Commitment through Self-Verification," *Social Psychology Quarterly* 62 (1999): 347–366; Stryker and Burke, "The Past, Present, and Future of Identity Theory."

20. See Sharon Hays, *Cultural Contradictions of Motherhood* (New Haven, CT: Yale University Press, 1996); Susan Douglas and Meredith Michaels, *The Mommy Myth* (New York: Free Press, 2004); Tiffany Taylor, "Re-examining Cultural Contradictions: Mothering Ideology and the Intersections of Class, Gender, and Race," *Sociology Compass* 5 (2011): 898–907; Lois, *Home Is Where the School Is*; Sarah Damaske, "Work, Family, and Accounts of Mothers' Lives Using Discourse to Navigate Intensive Mothering Ideals," *Sociology Compass* 7 (2013): 436–444.

21. Hays, *Cultural Contradictions of Motherhood*, 154.

22. Lois, *Home Is Where the School Is*.

23. Arlie Russell Hochschild, "Emotion Work, Feeling Rules, and Social Structure," *American Journal of Sociology* 85 (1979): 551–575.

24. Hochschild, "Emotion Work, Feeling Rules, and Social Structure"; Peggy A. Thoits, "Managing the Emotions of Others," *Symbolic Interaction* 19 (1996): 85–109.

25. Rebecca Erickson, "Reconceptualizing Family Work," *Journal of Marriage and Family* 55 (1993): 888–900; Scott Coltrane, "Research on Household Labor," *Journal of Marriage and Family* 62 (2000): 1208–1233; Rebecca Erickson, "Why Emotion Work Matters: Sex, Gender, and the Division of Household Labor," *Journal of Marriage and Family* 67 (2005): 337–351.

CHAPTER 6 DISRUPTED SELVES, MAKING SENSE, AND MAKING DO

1. Kenneth J. Gergen and Mary M. Gergen, "Narratives of the Self" in *Studies in Social Identity*, ed. Theodore R. Sarbin and Karl E. Scheibe (New York: Praeger, 1983), 254–273.

2. Sharon Hays, *Cultural Contradictions of Motherhood* (New Haven, CT: Yale University Press, 1996).

3. Kathleen Gerson, *Hard Choices: How Women Decide about Work, Career, and Motherhood* (Berkeley, CA: University of California Press, 1985); Kathleen Gerson, *No Man's Land: Men's Changing Commitments to Family and Work* (New York: Basic Books, 1993).

4. Mary Blair-Loy, *Competing Devotions: Career and Family Among Women Executives* (Cambridge, MA: Harvard University Press, 2003).

5. Gerson, *No Man's Land*, 141–181.

6. For a discussion of the temporal dimensions of identity, see Jenna Howard, "Expecting and Accepting: The Temporal Ambiguity of Recovery Identities," *Social Psychology Quarterly* 69 (2006): 307–324.

7. Jennifer Lois, "The Temporal Emotion Work of Motherhood: Homeschoolers' Strategies for Managing Time Shortage," *Gender & Society* 24 (2010): 421–446.

8. Philip Roth, *American Pastoral* (New York: Vintage Books, 1997).

9. Sandra Kumamoto Stanley, "Mourning the 'Greatest Generation': Myth and History in Philip Roth's American Pastoral," *Twentieth Century Literature* 15 (2005): 1–24.

10. Dennis P. Hogan and Nan Marie Astone, "The Transition to Adulthood," *Annual Review of Sociology* 12 (1986): 109–130.

11. Kellie J. Hagewen and S. Philip Morgan, "Intended and Ideal Family Size in the United States, 1970–2002." *Population and Development Review* 31 (2005): 507–527.

12. Erving Goffman, *Stigma: Notes on the Management of Spoiled Identity* (New York: Aronson, 1963); Bruce G. Link and Joe C. Phelan, "Conceptualizing Stigma," *Sociology* 27 (2001): 363–385.

13. Goffman, *Stigma*, 128.

14. Iain Wilkinson, *Suffering: A Sociological Introduction* (Cambridge: Polity Press, 2005), 55–68.

15. Emile Durkheim, *Suicide*, trans. John A. Spaulding and George Simpson (New York: The Free Press, 1966 [1897]).

16. Robert K. Merton, "Social Structure and Anomie," *American Sociological Review* 3 (1938): 672–682.

17. Ruohui Zhao and Liqun Cao, "Social Change and Anomie: A Cross-National Study," *Social Forces* 88 (2010): 1209–1230.

18. Wilkinson, *Suffering*, 71.

19. Peter Berger, *The Sacred Canopy: Elements of Sociological Theory of Religion* (Garden City, NY: Doubleday, 1967).

20. Ibid., 43.

21. Ibid., 43.

22. Ibid., 101, emphasis mine.

23. Arthur W. Frank, *The Wounded Storyteller: Body, Illness, and Ethics* (Chicago: University of Chicago Press, 1995), 75–96.

24. See Wilkinson, *Suffering*, 69–76.

25. Goffman, *Stigma.*

26. See also David Farrugia, "Exploring Stigma: Medical Knowledge and the Stigmatisation of Parents of Children Diagnosed with Autism Spectrum Disorder," *Sociology of Health & Illness* 31 (2009): 1011–1027.

27. The Parent Share is a pseudonym.

28. Elizabeth Kübler-Ross, *On Death and Dying* (New York: Simon and Schuster, 1969).

29. Emily Pearl Kingsley, "Welcome to Holland," in *Road Map to Holland: How I Found My Way Through My Son's First Two Years with Down Syndrome* by Jennifer Graf Groneberg (New York: New American Library, 2013), 291–292.

30. Frank, *The Wounded Storyteller*, 115–136.

31. Thomas DeGloma, "Awakenings: Autobiography, Memory, and the Social Logic of Personal Discovery," *Sociological Forum* 25 (2010): 519–540; Thomas DeGloma, *Seeing the Light: The Social Logic of Personal Discovery* (Chicago: University of Chicago Press, 2014).

32. Frank, *The Wounded Storyteller*, 75–96.

CHAPTER 7 FAMILY TROUBLE

1. C. Wright Mills, *The Sociological Imagination* (New York: Oxford University Press, 1959), 5 and 8.

2. James S. House, "The Three Faces of Social Psychology," *Sociometry* 40 (1977): 161–177; John F. Stolte, Gary Alan Fine, and Karen S. Cook, "Sociological Miniaturism: Seeing the Big through the Small in Social Psychology," *Annual Review of Sociology* 27 (2001): 387–413.

3. Sheldon Stryker and Peter J. Burke, "The Past, Present, and Future of Identity Theory," *Social Psychology Quarterly* 63 (2000): 284–297.

4. Anthony Giddens, *Modernity and Self-Identity: Self and Society in the Late Modern Age* (Cambridge: Polity Press, 1991); Anthony Giddens, *The Transformation of Intimacy* (Cambridge: Polity Press, 1992); Zygmunt Bauman, *Liquid Modernity* (Cambridge: Polity Press, 2000).

5. Jeffrey Jensen Arnette, "Emerging Adulthood: A Theory of Development from the Late Teens through the Twenties," *American Psychologist* 55 (2000): 469–480; John Bynner, "Rethinking the Youth Phase of the Life Course: The Case for Emerging Adulthood?" *Journal of Youth Studies* 8 (2005): 367–384.

6. Graham Allan, "Flexibility, Friendship, and Family," *Personal Relationships* 15 (2008): 3.

7. Arland Thornton and Linda Young-DeMarco, "Four Decades of Trends in Attitudes toward Family Issues in the United States: The 1960s through the 1990s," *Journal of Marriage and the Family* 63 (2001): 1009–1037; Jane Lewis, *The End of Marriage: Individualism and Intimate Relations* (Cheltenham: Edward Elgar, 2001); Judith A. Seltzer, "Cohabitation in the United States and Britain: Demography, Kinship, and the Future," *Journal of Marriage and Family* 66 (2004): 921–928; Tanya Koropeckyj-Cox and Gretchen Pendell, "Attitudes about Childlessness in the United States: Correlates of Positive, Neutral, and Negative Responses," *Journal of Family Issues* 28 (2007): 1054–1082.

8. Stephanie Coontz, *Marriage, A History: From Obedience to Intimacy, or How Love Conquered Marriage* (Berkeley, CA: University of California Press, 2005).

9. Kathleen Gerson, *The Unfinished Revolution: How a New Generation Is Reshaping Family, Work, and Gender in America* (New York: Oxford University Press, 2010).

10. See also Andrew J. Weigert and Ross Hastings, "Identity Loss, Family, and Social Change," *American Journal of Sociology* 82 (1977): 1171–1185.

11. For example, see Willard Waller, *The Old Love and the New* (New York: Horace Liveright, 1930); Fred Davis, *Passage through Crisis* (New York: Bobbs-Merrill, 1963); Diane Vaughan, *Uncoupling* (New York: Oxford University Press, 1986); Helena Znaniecka Lopata, *Current Widowhood* (Thousand Oaks, CA: Sage Publications, 1996); David A. Karp, *The Burden of Sympathy: How Families Cope with Mental Illness* (New York: Oxford University Press, 2001); Debra Umberson, *Death of a Parent: Transition to a New Adult Identity* (Cambridge: Cambridge University Press, 2003).

12. Vaughan, *Uncoupling*.

13. Ibid., 112 and 86.

14. Vaughan, *Uncoupling*; Catherine E. Ross, "Reconceptualizing Marital Status as a Continuum of Social Attachment," *Journal of Marriage and Family* 57 (1995): 129–140.

15. Vaughan, *Uncoupling*; Catherine Kohler Riessman, *Divorce Talk* (New Brunswick, NJ: Rutgers University Press, 1990); Theresa Arendell, *Fathers and Divorce* (Thousand Oaks, CA: Sage Publications, 1995).

16. Riessman, *Divorce Talk*.

17. Umberson, *Death of a Parent*, 7.

18. Harriet Engel Gross, "Couples Who Live Apart: Time/Place Disjunctions and Their Consequences," *Symbolic Interaction* 3 (1980): 73.

19. Beth Harry, "Making Sense of Disability: Low-Income, Puerto Rican Parents' Theories of the Problem," *Exceptional Children* 59 (1992): 27–40.

20. Vaughan, *Uncoupling*; Riessman, *Divorce Talk*; Debra Umberson and Meichu D. Chen, "Effects of a Parent's Death on Adult Children: Relationship Salience and Reaction to Loss," *American Sociological Review* 59 (1994): 152–168.

21. Sarah Wilson, "'When You Have Children, You're Obliged to Live': Motherhood, Chronic Illness, and Biographical Disruption," *Sociology of Health and Illness* 29 (2007): 610–626.

22. Erving Goffman, "The Insanity of Place," in *Relations in Public: Micro Studies of Public Order* (New York: Basic Books, 1971), 366.

23. See Robert M. Emerson and Sheldon L. Messinger, "The Micro-Politics of Trouble." *Social Problems* 25 (1977): 121–135.

24. Vaughan, *Uncoupling*.

25. Herbert Blumer, *Symbolic Interaction: Perspective and Method* (Berkeley, CA: University of California Press, 1969), 149–152.

26. Lillian B. Rubin, *Families on the Fault Line* (New York: Harper Collins Publishers, 1994).

27. Kai Erikson, *Everything in its Path* (New York: Simon and Schuster, 1976); Kai Erikson, *A New Species of Trouble: Explorations in Disaster, Trauma, and Community* (New York: W. W. Norton and Company Inc., 1994); Daina Cheyenne Harvey, "A Quiet Suffering: Some Notes on the Sociology of Suffering," *Sociological Forum* 27 (2012.): 528–535.

28. Giddens, *Modernity and Self-Identity*.

29. Peter Stearns, *Anxious Parents: A History of Modern Childrearing in America* (New York: New York University Press, 2003).

30. Simon J. Williams, "Chronic Illness as Biographical Disruption or Biographical Disruption as Chronic Illness? Reflections on a Core Concept," *Sociology of Health and Illness* 22 (2000): 40–67.

31. Allen V. Horwitz and Jerome C. Wakefield, *The Loss of Sadness: How Psychiatry Transformed Normal Sorrow into Depressive Disorder* (New York: Oxford University Press, 2007).

32. Ibid.

33. Ibid., 203.

34. Erich Goode, "Is the Sociology of Deviance Still Relevant?" *American Sociologist* 35 (2004): 46–57; Joel Best, "Deviance May Be Alive, But Is it Intellectually Lively? A Reaction to Goode," *Deviant Behavior* 25 (2004): 483–492; Patricia A. Adler and Peter Adler, "The Deviance Society," *Deviant Behavior* 27 (2006): 129–148.

APPENDIX A: METHODS

1. Andrew Solomon, *Far From the Tree: Parents, Children, and the Search for Identity* (New York: Scribner, 2012).

2. Arthur W. Frank, *The Wounded Storyteller: Body, Illness, and Ethics* (Chicago: University of Chicago Press, 1995).

3. Ibid.

4. Annette Lareau, *Unequal Childhoods: Class, Race and Family Life* (Berkeley, CA: University of California Press, 2003).

5. John Lofland, David Snow, Leon Anderson, and Lyn H. Lofland, *Analyzing Social Settings: A Guide To Qualitative Observation and Analysis* (Belmont: Wadsworth/Thomson Learning, 2006).

6. Even in cases of separation or divorce, I asked each participant if I could contact his or her child's other parent for an interview. Of the eighteen individuals whose counterparts did not participate, thirteen preferred that I not contact their children's other parents. In three cases, participants provided me with the necessary contact information, but their counterparts declined to participate. In the remaining two cases, one ex-spouse was deceased and the other did not live in the United States and was difficult to contact.

7. One participant identified all five of her adult children as having problems with drugs and alcohol, so while approximately one-third of children were over the age of eighteen, their parents represent a smaller fraction of participating mothers and fathers.

8. Lofland, Snow, Anderson, and Lofland, *Analyzing Social Settings: A Guide To Qualitative Observation and Analysis*, 105.

BIBLIOGRAPHY

Adamson, Christopher. "Existential and Clinical Uncertainty in the Medical Encounter: An Idiographic Account of an Illness Trajectory Defined by Inflammatory Bowel Disease and Avascular Necrosis." *Sociology of Health & Illness* 19 (1997): 133–159.

Adler, Patricia A., and Peter Adler. "The Deviance Society." *Deviant Behavior* 27 (2006): 129–148.

Allan, Graham. "Flexibility, Friendship, and Family." *Personal Relationships* 15 (2008): 1–16.

Appleton, Lynn M. "Rethinking Medicalization: Alcoholism and Anomalies." In *Images of Issues*, edited by Joel Best. Hawthorne, NY: Aldine de Gruyter, 1995: 59-80.

Arendell, Theresa. *Fathers and Divorce.* Thousand Oaks, CA: Sage Publications, 1995.

Ariès, Philippe. *Centuries of Childhood.* London: Jonathan Cape Ltd., 1962.

Arnette, Jeffrey Jensen. "Emerging Adulthood: A Theory of Development from the Late Teens through the Twenties." *American Psychologist* 55 (2000): 469–480.

Aron, Laudan, and Pamela Loprest. "Disability and the Education System." *Future of Children* 22 (2012): 97–122.

Bauman, Zygmunt. *Liquid Modernity.* Cambridge: Polity Press, 2000.

Beard, Renee L., and Patrick J. Fox. "Resisting Social Disenfranchisement: Negotiating Collective Identities and Everyday Life with Memory Loss." *Social Science & Medicine* 66 (2008): 1509–1520.

Becker, Gaylene. *Disrupted Lives: How People Create Meaning in a Chaotic World.* Berkeley, CA: University of California Press, 1997.

Berger, Peter L. *Invitation to Sociology: A Humanistic Perspective.* Garden City, NY: Doubleday, 1963.

———. *The Sacred Canopy: Elements of Sociological Theory of Religion.* Garden City, NY: Doubleday, 1967.

Berger, Peter L., and Hansfried Kellner. "Marriage and the Construction of Reality: A Contribution to the Microsociology of Knowledge." *Diogenes* 12 (1964): 1–24.

Best, Joel. "Deviance May Be Alive, but Is it Intellectually Lively? A Reaction to Goode." *Deviant Behavior* 25 (2004): 483–492.

Bianchi, Suzanne M. "Family Change and Time Allocation in American Families." *Annals of the American Academy of Political and Social Science* 638 (2011): 21–44.

Bianchi, Suzanne M., John P. Robinson, and Melissa A. Milkie. *Changing Rhythms of American Family Life.* New York: Russell Sage Foundation, 2006.

Birenbaum, Arnold. "On Managing Courtesy Stigma." *Journal of Health and Social Behavior* 11 (1970): 196–206.

Blair-Loy, Mary. *Competing Devotions: Career and Family among Women Executives.* Cambridge: Harvard University Press, 2003.

Blum, Linda. "Mother-Blame in the Prozac Nation: Raising Kids with Invisible Disabilities." *Gender & Society* 21 (2007): 202–226.

Blumer, Herbert. *Symbolic Interaction: Perspective and Method.* Berkeley, CA: University of California Press, 1969.

Blumstein, Philip. "The Production of Selves in Personal Relationships." In *The Self-Society Dynamic: Cognition, Emotional, and Action*, edited by Judith A. Howard and Peter L. Callero, 205–322. New York: Cambridge University Press, 1991.

Boss, Pauline. "Ambiguous Loss Research, Theory, and Practice." *Journal of Marriage and Family* 66 (2004): 551–566.

Bost, Kelly K., Martha J. Cox, and Chris Payne. "Structural and Supportive Changes in Couples' Family and Friendship Networks across the Transition to Parenthood." *Journal of Marriage and Family* 64 (2002): 517–531.

Brantlinger, Ellen. *Dividing Classes: How the Middle Class Negotiates and Rationalizes School Advantage.* New York: Routledge, 2003.

Burgard, Sarah A., and Jennifer A. Ailshire. "Gender and Time for Sleep among U.S. Adults." *American Sociological Review* 78 (2012): 51–69.

Burke, Peter J., and Donald C. Reitzes. "An Identity Theory Approach to Commitment." *Social Psychology Quarterly* 54 (1991): 239–251.

Burke, Peter J., and Jan E. Stets. "Trust and Commitment through Self-Verification." *Social Psychology Quarterly* 62 (1999): 347–366.

Bury, Michael. "Chronic Illness as Biographical Disruption." *Sociology of Health and Illness* 4 (1982): 167–182.

Butler, Judith. *Gender Trouble: Feminism and the Subversion of Identity.* New York: Routledge, 1990.

Bynner, John. "Rethinking the Youth Phase of the Life Course: The Case for Emerging Adulthood?" *Journal of Youth Studies* 8 (2005): 367–384.

Byrd, Robert, Allyson C. Sage, and Janet Keyzer. "Report to the Legislature on the Principal Findings of the Epidemiology of Autism in California: A Comprehensive Pilot Study." MIND Institute, 2002.

Byrne, Bridget. "In Search of a 'Good Mix': 'Race,' Class, Gender and Practices of Mothering." *Sociology* 40 (2006): 1001–1017.

Charmaz, Kathy. *Good Days, Bad Days.* New Brunswick, NJ: Rutgers University Press, 1991.

Charmaz, Kathy, and Melinda Milligan. "Grief." In *Handbook of the Sociology of Emotions,* edited by Jan E. Stets and Jonathan H. Turner, 516–543. New York: Springer, 2007.

Cheal, David. "Unity and Difference in Postmodern Families." *Journal of Family Issues* 14 (1993): 5–19.

Cherlin, Andrew J. "The Deinstitutionalization of American Marriage." *Journal of Marriage and Family* 66 (2004): 848–861.

Clarke, Candace. *Misery and Company: Sympathy in Everyday Life.* Chicago: University of Chicago Press, 1998.

Claxton, Amy, and Maureen Perry-Jenkins. "No Fun Anymore: Leisure and Marital Quality across the Transition to Parenthood." *Journal of Marriage and Family* 70 (2008): 28–43.

Coles, Gerald. *The Learning Mystique.* New York: Pantheon Books, 1987.

Coltrane, Scott. "Research on Household Labor." *Journal of Marriage and Family* 62 (2000): 1208–1233.

Conrad, Peter. "The Shifting Engines of Medicalization." *Journal of Health and Social Behavior* 46 (2005): 3–14.

———. *The Medicalization of Society: On the Transformation of Human Conditions into Treatable Disorders.* Baltimore: The Johns Hopkins University Press, 2007.

Conrad, Peter, and Joseph Schneider. *Deviance and Medicalization, From Badness to Sickness.* St. Louis: Mosby Publishing Company, 1980.

Coontz, Stephanie. *Marriage, A History: From Obedience to Intimacy, or How Love Conquered Marriage.* Berkeley, CA: University of California Press, 2005.

Corrigan, Patrick W., Amy C. Watson, and Fredrick E. Miller. "Blame, Shame, and Contamination: The Impact of Mental Illness and Drug Dependence Stigma on Family Members." *Journal of Family Psychology* 20 (2006): 239–246.

Craig, Lyn, and Killian Mullan. "Parenthood, Gender, and Work–Family Time in the United States, Australia, Italy, France, and Denmark." *Journal of Marriage and Family* 72 (2010): 1344–1361.

Damaske, Sarah. "Work, Family, and Accounts of Mothers' Lives Using Discourse to Navigate Intensive Mothering Ideals." *Sociology Compass* 7 (2013): 436–444.

Davis, Fred. *Passage through Crisis.* New York: Bobbs-Merrill, 1963.

Davis, Lennard J. *Enforcing Normalcy: Disability, Deafness, and the Body.* London: Verso, 1995.

DeGloma, Thomas. "Awakenings: Autobiography, Memory, and the Social Logic of Personal Discovery." *Sociological Forum* 25 (2010): 519–540.

———. *Seeing the Light: The Social Logic of Personal Discovery.* Chicago: University of Chicago Press, 2014.

Douglas, Susan, and Meredith Michaels. *The Mommy Myth.* New York: Free Press, 2004.

Durkheim, Emile. *Suicide.* Translated by John A. Spaulding and George Simpson. New York City: The Free Press, 1966 [1897].

Ebaugh, Helen Rose Fuchs. *Becoming an Ex: The Process of Role Exit.* Chicago: University of Chicago Press, 1988.

Edin, Kathryn, and Maria J. Kefalas. *Promises I Can Keep: Why Poor Women Put Motherhood Before Marriage.* Berkeley, CA: University of California Press, 2005.

Emerson, Robert M. "Responding to Roommate Troubles: Reconsidering Informal Dyadic Control." *Law & Society Review* 42 (2008): 483–512.

———. "Ethnography, Interaction, and Ordinary Trouble." *Ethnography* 10 (2009): 535–548.

———. "From Normal Conflict to Normative Deviance: The Micro-Politics of Trouble in Close Relationships." *Journal of Contemporary Ethnography* 40 (2011): 3–38.

Emerson, Robert M., and Sheldon L. Messinger. "The Micro-Politics of Trouble." *Social Problems* 25 (1977): 121–135.

Erickson, Rebecca. "Reconceptualizing Family Work." *Journal of Marriage and Family* 55 (1995): 888–900.

———. "Why Emotion Work Matters: Sex, Gender, and the Division of Household Labor." *Journal of Marriage and Family* 67 (2005): 337–351.

Erikson, Kai. *Everything in Its Path.* New York: Simon and Schuster, 1976.

———. *A New Species of Trouble: Explorations in Disaster, Trauma, and Community.* New York: W. W. Norton, 1994.

Farrugia, David. "Exploring Stigma: Medical Knowledge and the Stigmatisation of Parents of Children Diagnosed with Autism Spectrum Disorder." *Sociology of Health & Illness* 31 (2009): 1011–1027.

Frank, Arthur W. *Wounded Storyteller: Body, Illness, and Ethics.* Chicago: University of Chicago Press, 1995.

Fox, Renee C. "Medical Uncertainty Revisited." In *The Handbook of Social Studies in Health and Medicine,* edited by Gary L. Albrecht, Ray Fitzpatrick, and Susan C. Scrimshaw, 409–425. London: Sage, 2000.

Gallagher, Sally K., and Naomi Gerstel. "Connections and Constraints: The Effects of Children on Caregiving." *Journal of Marriage and the Family* 63 (2001): 265–275.

Garey, Anita, and Terry Arendell. "Children, Work, and Family: Some Thoughts on 'Mother-Blame.'" In *Working Families: The Transformation of the American Home,* edited by Rosanna Hertz and Nancy Marshall, 293–303. Berkeley, CA: University of California Press, 2001.

Garfinkel, Harold. "Studies of the Routine Grounds of Everyday Activities." *Social Problems* 11 (1964): 225–250.

Gergen, Kenneth J., and Mary M. Gergen. "Narratives of the Self." In *Studies in Social Identity*, edited by Theodore R. Sarbin and Karl E. Scheibe, 254–273. New York: Praeger, 1983.

Gerson, Kathleen. *Hard Choices: How Women Decide about Work, Career, and Motherhood.* Berkeley, CA: University of California Press, 1985.

———. *No Man's Land: Men's Changing Commitments to Family and Work.* New York: Basic Books, 1993.

———. *The Unfinished Revolution: How a New Generation Is Reshaping Family, Work, and Gender in America.* New York: Oxford University Press, 2010.

Giddens, Anthony. *Modernity and Self-Identity: Self and Society in the Late Modern Age.* Cambridge: Polity Press, 1991.

———. *The Transformation of Intimacy.* Cambridge: Polity Press, 1992.

Gillis, John R. *A World of Their Own Making.* Cambridge, MA: Harvard University Press, 1996.

Goffman, Erving. *Stigma: Notes on the Management of Spoiled Identity.* New York: Aronson, 1963.

———. "The Insanity of Place." In *Relations in Public: Microstudies of Public Order*, 335–390. New York: Basic Books, 1971.

Golden, Janet. *Message in a Bottle.* Cambridge, MA: Harvard University Press, 2005.

Goode, Erich. "Is the Sociology of Deviance Still Relevant?" *American Sociologist* 35 (2004): 46–57.

Gray, David. "High Functioning Autistic Children and the Construction of 'Normal' Family Life." *Social Science and Medicine* 44 (1997): 1097–1106.

———. "'Everybody Just Freezes. Everybody Is Just Embarrassed': Felt and Enacted Stigma among Parents of Children with High Functioning Autism." *Sociology of Health and Illness* 24 (2002): 734–749.

Green, Sara E. "'Oh, Those Therapists Will Become Your Best Friends': Maternal Satisfaction with Clinics Providing Physical, Occupational, and Speech Therapy Services to Children with Disabilities." *Sociology of Health & Illness* 23 (2001): 798–828.

———. "What Do You Mean 'What's Wrong With Her?': Stigma and the Lives of Families of Children with Disabilities." *Social Science & Medicine* 57 (2003): 1361–1374.

———. "The Impact of Stigma on Maternal Attitudes toward Placement of Children with Disabilities in Residential Care Facilities." *Social Science & Medicine* 59 (2004): 799–812.

Green, Sara E., Christine Davis, Elana Karshmer, Pete Marsh, and Benjamin Straight. "Living Stigma: The Impact of Labeling, Stereotyping, Separation, Status Loss, and Discrimination in the Lives of Individuals with Disabilities and Their Families." *Sociological Inquiry* 75 (2005): 197–215.

Gross, Edward, and Gregory P. Stone. "Embarrassment and the Analysis of Role Requirements." *American Journal of Sociology* 70 (1964): 1–15.

Gross, Harriet Engel. "Couples Who Live Apart: Time/Place Disjunctions and Their Consequences." *Symbolic Interaction* 3 (1980): 69–82.

Hagewen, Kellie J., and S. Philip Morgan. "Intended and Ideal Family Size in the United States, 1970–2002." *Population and Development Review* 31 (2005): 507–527.

Hallowell, Nina, Audrey Arden-Jones, Ros Eeles, Claire Foster, Anneke Lucassen, Clare Moynihan, and Maggie Watson. "Guilt, Blame and Responsibility: Men's Understanding of Their Role in the Transmission of BRCA1/2 Mutations Within Their Family." *Sociology of Health & Illness* 28 (2006): 969–988.

Hankiss, Agnes. "Ontologies of the Self: On the Mythological Rearranging of One's Life History." In *Biography and Society: The Life History Approach in the Social Sciences*, edited by Daniel Bertaux, 203–209. Los Angeles, CA: Sage Publications, 1981.

Hareven, Tamara K. *Families, History, and Social Change: Life Course and Cross Cultural Perspectives.* Boulder, CO: Westview Press, 2000.

Harry, Beth. "Making Sense of Disability: Low-Income, Puerto Rican Parents' Theories of the Problem." *Exceptional Children* 59 (1992): 27–40.

Harvey, Daina Cheyenne. "A Quiet Suffering: Some Notes on the Sociology of Suffering." *Sociological Forum* 27 (2012): 528–535.

Hays, Sharon. *Cultural Contradictions of Motherhood.* New Haven, CT: Yale University Press, 1996.

Hochschild, Arlie Russell. "Emotion Work, Feeling Rules, and Social Structure." *American Journal of Sociology* 85 (1979): 551–575.

Hogan, Dennis P., and Nan Marie Astone. "The Transition to Adulthood." *Annual Review of Sociology* 12 (1986): 109–130.

Holstein, James A., and Jaber F. Gubrium. "Deprivatization and the Construction of Domestic Life." *Journal of Marriage and the Family* 57 (1995): 894–908.

Horn, Wade F., and Douglas Tynan. "Revamping Special Education." *Public Interest* 114 (2001): 36–53.

Horwitz, Allan V., and Jerome C. Wakefield. *The Loss of Sadness: How Psychiatry Transformed Normal Sorrow into Depressive Disorder.* New York: Oxford University Press, 2007.

House, James S. "The Three Faces of Social Psychology." *Sociometry* 40 (1977): 161–177.

Howard, Jenna. "Expecting and Accepting: The Temporal Ambiguity of Recovery Identities." *Social Psychology Quarterly* 69 (2006): 307–324.

Hughes, Everett C. "Dilemmas and Contradictions of Status." *American Journal of Sociology* 50 (1945): 353–359.

Ishii-Kuntz, Masako, and Karen Seccombe. "The Impact of Children upon Social Support Networks Throughout the Life Course." *Journal of Marriage and the Family* 51 (1989): 777–790.

Jefferson, Gail. "On 'Trouble-Premonitory' Response to Inquiry." *Sociological Inquiry* 50 (1980): 153–185.

Karp, David A. *Speaking of Sadness: Depression, Disconnection, and the Meanings of Illness.* New York: Oxford University Press, 1997.

———. *The Burden of Sympathy: How Families Cope with Mental Illness.* New York: Oxford University Press, 2001.

Kessler-Harris, Alice. *Out to Work: A History of Wage-Earning Women in the United States.* New York: Oxford University Press, 2003.

Kidder-Ashley, Pamela, James R. Deni, and Jessica B. Anderton. "Learning Disabilities Eligibility in the 1990s: Analysis of State Practices." *Education* 121 (2000): 65–73.

Kingsley, Emily Pearl. "Welcome to Holland." In *Road Map to Holland: How I Found My Way Through My Son's First Two Years with Down Syndrome* by Jennifer Graf Groneberg, 291–292. New York: New American Library, 2013.

Knudsen, Knud, and Kari Wærness. "National Context and Spouses' Housework in 34 Countries." *European Sociological Review* 24 (2008): 97–113.

Koro-Ljungberg, Mirka, and Regina Bussing. "The Management of Courtesy Stigma in the Lives of Families with Teenagers with ADHD." *Journal of Family Issues* 30 (2009): 1175–2000.

Koropeckyj-Cox, Tanya, and Gretchen Pendell. "Attitudes about Childlessness in the United States: Correlates of Positive, Neutral, and Negative Responses." *Journal of Family Issues* 28 (2007): 1054–1082.

Kübler-Ross, Elizabeth. *On Death and Dying.* New York: Simon and Schuster, 1969.

Ladd-Taylor, Molly, and Lauri Umansky, eds. *"Bad" Mothers: The Politics of Blame in Twentieth Century America*. New York: New York University Press, 1998.

Lareau, Annette. *Unequal Childhoods: Class, Race and Family Life*. Berkeley, CA: University of California Press, 2003.

Lewis, Jane. *The End of Marriage: Individualism and Intimate Relations*. Cheltenham: Edward Elgar, 2001.

Link, Bruce G., and Joe C. Phelan. "Conceptualizing Stigma." *Annual Review of Sociology* 27 (2001): 363–385.

Litt, Jacquelyn. "Women's Carework in Low-Income Households: The Special Case of Children with Attention Deficit Hyperactivity Disorder." *Gender & Society* 18 (2004): 625–644.

Lofland, John, David Snow, Leon Anderson, and Lyn H. Lofland. *Analyzing Social Settings: A Guide to Qualitative Observation and Analysis*. Belmont: Wadsworth/Thomson Learning, 2006.

Lofland, Lyn H. "Loss and Human Connection: An Exploration into the Nature of the Social Bond." In *Personality, Roles, and Social Behavior*, edited by William Ickes and Eric S. Knowles, 219–242. New York: Springer-Verlag, 1982.

Lois, Jennifer. "The Temporal Emotion Work of Motherhood: Homeschoolers' Strategies for Managing Time Shortage." *Gender & Society* 24 (2010): 421–446.

———. *Home Is Where the School Is: The Logic of Homeschooling and the Emotional Labor of Mothering*. New York: New York University Press, 2012.

Lopata, Helena Znaniecka. *Current Widowhood*. Thousand Oaks, CA: Sage Publications, 1996.

Mahoney, Annette, Kenneth I. Pargament, Aaron Murray-Swank, and Nichole Murray-Swank. "Religion and the Sanctification of Family Relationships." *Review of Religious Research* 44 (2003): 220–236.

Maines, David R. *The Faultline of Consciousness: A View of Interactionism in Sociology*. New York: Aldine De Gruyter, 2001.

Malacrida, Claudia. *Cold Comfort: Mothers, Professionals, and Attention Deficit (Hyperactivity) Disorder*. Toronto: University of Toronto Press, 2003.

———. "Medicalization, Ambivalence and Social Control: Mothers' Descriptions of Educators and ADD/ADHD." In *Health: An Interdisciplinary Journal for the Social Study of Health, Illness and Medicine* 8 (2004): 61–80.

Martin, Jack K., Bernice A. Pescosolido, Sigrun Olafsdottir, and Jane D. McLeod. "The Construction of Fear: Americans' Preferences for Social Distance from Children and Adolescents with Mental Health Problems." *Journal of Health and Social Behavior* 48 (2007): 50–67.

May, Carl. "Pathology, Identity and the Social Construction of Alcohol Dependence." *Sociology* 35 (2001): 385–401.

Mead, George Herbert. *Mind, Self, and Society*. Chicago: University of Chicago Press, 1934.

Mercer, Jane R. "Social System Perspective and Clinical Perspective: Frames of Reference for Understanding Career Patterns of Persons Labeled as Mental Retarded." *Social Problems* 13 (1965): 18–34.

Merton, Robert K. "Social Structure and Anomie." *American Sociological Review* 3 (1938): 672–682.

Mickelson, Kristin D. "Perceived Stigma, Social Support, and Depression." *Personality and Social Psychology Bulletin* 27 (2001): 1046–1056.

Milkie, Melissa A., Suzanne M. Bianchi, Marybeth J. Mattingly, and John P. Robinson. "Gendered Division of Childrearing: Ideals, Realities, and the Relationship to Parental Well-Being." *Sex Roles* 47 (2002): 21–38.

Mills, C. Wright. *The Sociological Imagination*. New York: Oxford University Press, 1959.

Oliver, Michael. *The Politics of Disablement: A Sociological Approach*. London: Palgrave Macmillan, 1990.

Pugh, Allison. *Longing and Belonging: Parents, Children, and Consumer Culture*. Berkeley, CA: University of California Press, 2009.

Rafalovich, Adam. "Attention Deficit-Hyperactivity Disorder as the Medicalization of Childhood: Challenges from and for Sociology." *Sociology Compass* 7 (2013): 343–354.

Riessman, Catherine Kohler. *Divorce Talk*. New Brunswick, NJ: Rutgers University Press, 1990.

Rosenberg, Charles, and Janet Golden. *Framing Disease: Studies in Cultural History*. New Brunswick, NJ: Rutgers University Press, 1992.

Ross, Catherine E. "Reconceptualizing Marital Status as a Continuum of Social Attachment." *Journal of Marriage and Family* 57 (1995): 129–140.

Roth, Philip. *American Pastoral*. New York: Vintage Books, 1997.

Rubin, Lillian B. *Families on the Fault Line*. New York: Harper Collins Publishers, 1994.

Scambler, Graham, and Anthony Hopkins. "Being Epileptic: Coming to Terms with Stigma." *Sociology of Health and Illness* 8 (1986): 26–43.

Seltzer, Judith A. "Cohabitation in the United States and Britain: Demography, Kinship, and the Future." *Journal of Marriage and Family* 66 (2004): 921–928.

Shirani, Fiona, Karen Henwood, and Carrie Coltart. "Meeting the Challenges of Intensive Parenting Culture: Gender, Risk, Management and the Moral Parent." *Sociology* 46 (2012): 25–40.

Simon, Robin W. "The Joys of Parenthood, Reconsidered." *Contexts* 7 (2008): 40–45.

Singh, Ilina. "Boys Will Be Boys: Fathers' Perspectives on ADHD Symptoms, Diagnosis and Drug Treatment." *Harvard Review of Psychiatry* 11 (2003): 308–316.

———. "Doing Their Jobs: Mothering with Ritalin in a Culture of Mother-Blame." *Social Science and Medicine* 59 (2004): 1193–1205.

Smith, Dorothy E. "The Standard North American Family: SNAF as an Ideological Code." *Journal of Family Issues* 14 (1993): 50–65.

Snow, David A., and Leon Anderson. *Down on Their Luck: A Study of Homeless Street People*. Berkeley, CA: University of California Press, 1993.

Solomon, Andrew. *Far From the Tree*. New York: Scribner, 2012.

Stanley, Sandra Kumamoto. "Mourning the 'Greatest Generation': Myth and History in Philip Roth's *American Pastoral*." *Twentieth Century Literature* Spring (2005): 1–24.

Stearns, Peter. *Anxious Parents: A History of Modern Childrearing in America*. New York: New York University Press, 2003.

Stockl, Andrea. "Complex Syndromes, Ambivalent Diagnosis, and Existential Uncertainty: The Case of Systemic Lupus Erythematosus (SLE)." *Social Science & Medicine* 65 (2007): 1549–1559.

Stolte, John F., Gary Alan Fine, and Karen S. Cook. "Sociological Miniaturism: Seeing the Big through the Small in Social Psychology." *Annual Review of Sociology* 27 (2001): 387–413.

Strauss, Anselm. *Mirrors and Masks*. Glencoe: Free Press, 1959.

Stryker, Sheldon, and Peter J. Burke. "The Past, Present, and Future of Identity Theory." *Social Psychology Quarterly* 63 (2000): 284–297.

Swain, John, Sally French, Colin Barnes, and Carol Thomas, eds. *Disabling Barriers, Enabling Environments*. London: Sage, 2004.

Szalavitz, Maia. *Help at Any Cost: How the Troubled-Teen Industry Cons Parents and Hurts Kids.* London: Penguin Books, 2006.

Taylor, Tiffany. "Re-examining Cultural Contradictions: Mothering Ideology and the Intersections of Class, Gender, and Race." *Sociology Compass* 5 (2011): 898–907.

Thoits, Peggy A. "Managing the Emotions of Others." *Symbolic Interaction* 19 (1996): 85–109.

Thornton, Arland, and Linda Young-DeMarco. "Four Decades of Trends in Attitudes toward Family Issues in the United States: The 1960s through the 1990s." *Journal of Marriage and the Family* 63 (2001): 1009–1037.

Thurer, Shari L. *The Myths of Motherhood: How Culture Reinvents the Good Mother.* Boston: Houghton Mifflin Company, 1994.

Umberson, Debra. *Death of a Parent: Transition to a New Adult Identity.* Cambridge: Cambridge University Press, 2003.

Umberson, Debra, and Meichu D. Chen. "Effects of a Parent's Death on Adult Children: Relationship Salience and Reaction to Loss." *American Sociological Review* 59 (1994): 152–168.

Vaughan, Diane. *Uncoupling.* New York: Oxford University Press, 1986.

Waite, Linda J., and Mark Nielsen. "The Rise of the Dual-Worker Family: 1963–1997." In *Working Families: The Transformation of the American Home*, edited by Rosanna Hertz and Nancy L. Marshall, 23–41. Berkeley, CA: University of California Press. 2001.

Waller, Willard. *The Old Love and the New.* New York: Horace Liveright, 1930.

Warner, Judith. *Perfect Madness: Motherhood in the Age of Anxiety.* New York: Riverhead Books, 2005.

Weigert, Andrew J., and Ross Hastings. "Identity Loss, Family, and Social Change." *American Journal of Sociology* 82 (1977): 1171–1185.

Wilkinson, Iain. *Suffering: A Sociological Introduction.* Cambridge: Polity Press, 2005.

Williams, Simon J. "Chronic Illness as Biographical Disruption or Biographical Disruption as Chronic Illness? Reflections on a Core Concept." *Sociology of Health and Illness* 22 (2000): 40–67.

Wilson, Sarah. "'When You Have Children, You're Obliged to Live': Motherhood, Chronic Illness, and Biographical Disruption." *Sociology of Health and Illness* 29 (2007): 610–626.

Wolf, Joan B. *Is Breast Best?: Taking on the Breastfeeding Experts and the New High Stakes of Motherhood.* New York: New York University Press, 2011.

Young, Bridget, Mary Dixon-Woods, Michelle Findlay, and David Heney. "Parenting in a Crisis: Conceptualising Mothers of Children with Cancer." *Social Science & Medicine* 55 (2002): 1835–1847.

Zelizer, Viviana A. *Pricing the Priceless Child: The Changing Social Value of Children.* Princeton, NJ: Princeton University Press, 1985.

Zerubavel, Eviatar. *Hidden Rhythms: Schedules and Calendars in Social Life.* Chicago: University of Chicago Press, 1981.

———. *Time Maps: Collective Memory and the Social Shape of the Past.* Chicago: University of Chicago Press, 2003.

———. "Generally Speaking: The Logic and Mechanics of Social Pattern Analysis." *Sociological Forum* 22 (2007): 131–145.

Zhao, Ruohui, and Liqun Cao. "Social Change and Anomie: A Cross-National Study." *Social Forces* 88 (2010): 1209–1230.

INDEX

ABOUT THE AUTHOR

ARA FRANCIS is an assistant professor of sociology at the College of the Holy Cross where she teaches courses in micro-sociology, deviance, and social disruption. She earned her PhD in sociology from the University of California, Davis.

CPSIA information can be obtained
at www.ICGtesting.com
Printed in the USA
FFOW01n1436280416
23665FF